SBA and MTF MCQs for the Primary FRCA

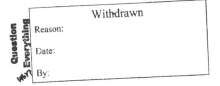

SBA and MTF MCQs for the Primary FRCA

The FRCAQ Writers Group

The Severn Deanery

Dr James Nickells
North Bristol NHS Trust

Dr Benjamin Walton
North Bristol NHS Trust

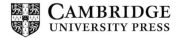
CAMBRIDGE
UNIVERSITY PRESS

CAMBRIDGE UNIVERSITY PRESS
Cambridge, New York, Melbourne, Madrid, Cape Town,
Singapore, São Paulo, Delhi, Mexico City

Cambridge University Press
The Edinburgh Building, Cambridge CB2 8RU, UK

Published in the United States of America by Cambridge University Press, New York

www.cambridge.org
Information on this title: www.cambridge.org/9781107604063

First published 2012

Printed in the United Kingdom at the University Press, Cambridge

A catalogue record for this publication is available from the British Library

Library of Congress Cataloguing in Publication data
Nickells, James.
SBA and MTF MCQs for the primary FRCA / James Nickells, Ben Walton.
   p.   cm.
ISBN 978-1-107-60406-3 (pbk.)
1. Anesthesia – Examinations, questions, etc.   I. Walton, Benjamin.   II. Title.
RD82.3.N529   2012
617.9'6076–dc23
                                                                2011049748
ISBN 978-1-10760406-3 Paperback

Contents

Contributors

DR EMMA BELLCHAMBERS Trainee, Severn Deanery, Bristol, UK

DR PHILIP M. BEWLEY Trainee, Severn Deanery, Bristol, UK

DR TIM BOWLES Trainee, Severn Deanery, Bristol, UK

DR HELEN CAIN Trainee, Severn Deanery, Bristol, UK

DR TOBIAS EVERETT Trainee, Severn Deanery, Bristol, UK

DR DAN FRESHWATER-TURNER Trainee, Severn Deanery, Bristol, UK

DR ANDY GEORGIOU Trainee, Severn Deanery, Bristol, UK

DR SIOBHAN KING Trainee, Severn Deanery, Bristol, UK

DR SOPHIE MACDOUGALL-DAVIES Trainee, Severn Deanery, Bristol, UK

DR HENRY MURDOCH Trainee, Severn Deanery, Bristol, UK

DR JAMES NICKELLS Consultant Anaesthetist, North Bristol NHS Trust, Bristol, UK

DR SONJA PAYNE Trainee, Severn Deanery, Bristol, UK

DR ANNABEL PEARSON Trainee, Severn Deanery, Bristol, UK

DR HELEN TURNHAM Trainee, Severn Deanery, Bristol, UK

DR BENJAMIN WALTON Consultant in Critical Care and Anaesthesia, North Bristol NHS Trust, Bristol, UK

Preface

By the time you have started revising for the Primary FRCA two things are true, namely that you will have taken (and passed) a fair number of exams and also that you will have developed a way of revising that works best for you. When we took the Primary FRCA there were a number of revision aids available to us including text-books, MCQ books, past questions that were surreptitiously passed from person to person and any number of revision courses, depending on how wealthy or nervous you were feeling. Most of our peers utilised various combinations of the above, but it would be fair to say that, at some point, MCQ books featured in everybody's plans. Since then the World Wide Web has appeared – and this has given another option that is rapidly growing in popularity, with a number of websites offering banks of questions that purport to be an accurate reflection of those contained within the exam. Some offer some explanation to go with them and others just the answers. The reasons for the growth in popularity of the Web as a revision aid are multi-factorial. The Web allows large volumes of material to be accessed and utilised in a far more dynamic way than content contained in books. This material is easier to update, and analysis of performance compared to other candidates is also possible. On a good website, candidates can also feed back comments about questions, which can then be altered if appropriate.

We believe that the Web will play an increasingly important part in exam revision, which is why, in conjunction with Cambridge University Press, we have developed FRCAQ.com. This is a bespoke site for candidates attempting both the Primary and Final FRCA examination. Contained within it is a mixture of multiple true false (MTF) and single best answer (SBA) MCQ questions. All the questions are written in a similar style to those contained within the exam and each is accompanied by both a short and a long explanation. The questions cover every aspect of the published College syllabus and are constantly reviewed and updated.

This book contains 180 questions from the website, allowing both a taster of the full website content and also a different way of learning that will suit some people's working patterns and preferences and allow people to still work when internet reception is poor!

We hope you will enjoy this book, and we trust that both it and the website will help you pass the exam with flying colours!

The College exam

At time of writing the MCQ component of the Primary FRCA exam consists of 90 MCQ questions. 60 of these are MTF and 30 are SBA, the latter first appearing in the September 2010 exam. The 30 SBA questions are made up of 20 in clinical anaesthesia, 5 in intensive care medicine and 5 in pain management. There is no negative marking, so our all-encompassing and incisive exam technique advice is "read each question carefully and answer them all"! The MTF questions are there to test theoretical knowledge and factual recall, whereas the SBA questions are designed to test the ability of the candidate to process and apply this knowledge. SBAs also help to spread the range of marks in an exam, and in the absence of negative marking they reduce the power of pure guesswork.

One needs to employ a different technique when answering an SBA question compared to an MTF. A good SBA question should contain more than one answer where you are left thinking "well, that's possible" or words to that effect. Therefore you must read each answer carefully before deciding on the best option. It is very unlikely that all answers will sound equally plausible, so it should be possible to eliminate one or two of the options, even if deciding between those that remain will involve an element of guesswork.

James Nickells and Benjamin Walton
on behalf of the FRCAQ.com writing team

Question Papers

Paper 1

MTF Question 1

Which of the following statements regarding logarithms are true?

(a) $pH = \log_{10} [H^+]$
(b) A solution with a pH of 6 is twice as alkaline as a solution with a pH of 3
(c) A solution with a pH of 3 has 1/100th the acidity of a solution with a pH of 5
(d) An acid with an H^+ concentration of 0.0001 M has a pH of 3
(e) A solution with a pH of 8 is 100 times more acidic than a solution with a pH of 10

MTF Question 2

Which of the following statements about etomidate are true?

(a) The standard induction dose of etomidate is 0.3 mg/kg
(b) Etomidate owes its anaesthetic activity to its action as an NMDA receptor antagonist
(c) Etomidate is not suitable for use in major trauma since it raises intracranial pressure
(d) Etomidate reversibly blocks the activity of the adrenocortical hormone 11β-hydroxylase
(e) Etomidate has intrinsic analgesic activity equivalent to 5–10 mg of intravenous morphine

MTF Question 3

Which of the following are required methods for testing medical gas cylinders in the UK?

(a) Hydrostatic testing
(b) Impact testing
(c) Internal visual inspection
(d) Ultrasonic testing
(e) Tensile strength testing

MTF Question 4

Regarding sodium in the human body, which of the following statements are true?

(a) Sodium is key to the cellular co-transport (symport) or counter-transport (antiport) of virtually every other ion

(b) It has a marginally higher concentration in cerebrospinal fluid than in plasma
(c) Its Nernst potential is about −60 mV
(d) Membrane-bound Na^+/K^+-ATPase extrudes three sodium ions for every two potassium ions that are taken up
(e) Adult kidneys filter 25 mol of sodium a day

MTF Question 5

Heparin-induced thrombocytopenia (HIT):

(a) Is likely to require platelet transfusion
(b) Usually presents with haemorrhage
(c) Is mediated via an IgG autoantibody combined with platelet factor 4
(d) Is most common with bovine heparin
(e) Usually takes 36 hours to develop following a patient's first exposure to heparin

MTF Question 6

Which of the following statements regarding mathematical concepts about relationships and graphs are true?

(a) In a multi-compartment pharmacokinetic model, drug can only be eliminated from the central compartment
(b) A bi-exponential decline is seen in two-compartment models
(c) Mammillary models have peripheral compartments that are directly linked to each other
(d) The rate of transfer from the central compartment to a peripheral compartment is constant
(e) In a multi-compartment pharmacokinetic model, a 'vessel-rich' peripheral compartment is where anaesthetic drugs have their effect

MTF Question 7

Regarding the code used to classify artificial cardiac pacemakers, which of the following are correct?

(a) The first letter denotes the chamber paced
(b) The second letter denotes the chamber paced
(c) The first letter denotes the chamber in which electrical activity is sensed
(d) The third letter represents rate modulation
(e) The fourth letter represents rate modulation

MTF Question 8

Regarding diathermy, which of the following are true?

(a) The current density at the patient plate or neutral electrode is relatively low in monopolar diathermy
(b) Monopolar diathermy is safer than unipolar diathermy for patients with cardiac pacemakers
(c) Alternating current at frequencies between 0.5 and 1 MHz is used
(d) The high frequencies used penetrate the myocardium
(e) The amount of heat generated by diathermy is proportional to the square of the current divided by the area

MTF Question 9

Regarding changes to the body that occur with ageing and might affect pharmacology:

(a) Decrease in opioid receptor numbers and increase in receptor affinity are the main causes of toxicity due to opioids in the elderly
(b) Reduced muscle bulk results in a prolonged effect for remifentanil
(c) Bioavailability of drugs absorbed by the gastrointestinal system decreases by 50% by the age of 80 years old
(d) As you age, you develop a relative decrease in body fat
(e) As you age your volume of distribution (V_D) for water-soluble drugs decreases

MTF Question 10

Regarding cellular metabolism, which of the following statements are correct?

(a) Aerobic metabolism of glucose is 80% efficient
(b) 1 mol of glucose yields 38 mol of adenosine triphosphate (ATP) under aerobic conditions
(c) The hexose monophosphate shunt produces carbon dioxide, ribose-5-phosphate and ATP
(d) Glycogen is stored in skeletal muscle and the liver in approximately equal proportions
(e) Under aerobic and anaerobic conditions, glycolysis generates a net gain of two ATP and two NADH

MTF Question 11

Regarding the adrenal glands, which of the following are true?

(a) The adrenal glands are retroperitoneal structures
(b) The adrenal cortex develops from mesoderm
(c) ACTH activates receptors in the zona fasciculata and the zona reticularis
(d) The inner adrenal cortex produces the glucocorticoids
(e) The adrenal glands are located inferior to the kidneys

MTF Question 12

Regarding infrared radiation:

(a) Radiation is the most important route for heat loss from the body during anaesthesia
(b) Radiation cannot transfer heat between two objects unless they are in contact with each other
(c) Reflective shiny metallised plastic foil blankets should be used in theatre to prevent heat loss from radiation
(d) Vasodilation increases heat loss by radiation
(e) Radiation accounts for up to 50% of normal heat loss from the body

MTF Question 13

As an antiemetic, dexamethasone:

(a) Is an effective rescue agent for postoperative vomiting
(b) Should be administered at the beginning of the surgery
(c) Is contraindicated for use in children

(d) Should be used intraoperatively as an antiemetic with caution because of an increased risk of immunosuppression and wound infection
(e) If given to an awake patient may produce uncomfortable perineal sensations

MTF Question 14

Regarding the use of drugs in pregnant women, which of the following agents are tocolytic?

(a) Inhaled isoflurane
(b) Intrathecal opioids
(c) Intravenous glyceryl trinitrate
(d) Intravenous magnesium sulphate
(e) Epidural bupivacaine

MTF Question 15

Which of the following are correct in relation to the Doppler effect?

(a) The Doppler effect describes the phenomenon by which the amplitude of sound waves is altered if the source is moving in relation to the detector
(b) The amplitude of sound waves is increased if the source of the sound is moving towards the detector
(c) The frequency of sound waves is reduced if the source of the sound is moving away from the detector
(d) The Doppler effect is used to measure blood flow velocity in arteries
(e) The Doppler effect is used in obstetric practice when a fetal heart rate monitor is used

MTF Question 16

Regarding the mechanism of secondary hyperalgesia:

(a) Dorsal horn cells show reduced excitability in response to persistent pain
(b) Excitation thresholds for mechanical stimuli in the dorsal horn cells fall
(c) An increased area of receptive afferent input can be demonstrated
(d) Secondary hyperalgesia is primarily due to a neuroplastic response in the dorsal horn
(e) The presence of magnesium ions enhances the activity of NMDA receptors

MTF Question 17

Which of the following statements are true regarding laryngoscope blades?

(a) The standard Macintosh laryngoscope blade is available in four sizes
(b) The Magill laryngoscope blade is curved
(c) The Macintosh laryngoscope blade should be placed anterior to the epiglottis in the vallecula during laryngoscopy for intubation
(d) The Miller laryngoscope blade should be placed anterior to the epiglottis in the vallecula during laryngoscopy for intubation
(e) A 'left-sided' version of the Macintosh laryngoscope blade is available

MTF Question 18

Regarding narcotic analgesia in children:

(a) An 8-year-old child may be prescribed a patient-controlled analgesia (PCA) device
(b) Parent-controlled analgesia (PrCA) is rarely used because it is likely to produce apnoea or excessive narcosis

(c) Neonates do not require opioids

(d) All children under 10 years old receiving an opioid infusion should have continuously monitored pulse oximetry

(e) Nasal fentanyl is not recommended in children under the age of 10 because of the risk of apnoea

MTF Question 19

Which of the following statements regarding the measurement of cardiac output using thermodilution are correct?

(a) The cold solution should be injected into the right ventricle

(b) Injection is performed during the inspiratory phase of the breathing cycle

(c) The graphical data obtained has temperature increasing on the y axis

(d) Semi-logarithmic data is required for the calculation of cardiac output

(e) The cardiac output is the area under the temperature–time graph

MTF Question 20

Regarding insulin:

(a) Some intermediate-acting insulins should not be used in patients with known allergy to heparin

(b) The majority of insulin used in the UK is structurally human insulin

(c) Complexing insulin with zinc decreases the rate at which it is absorbed

(d) 50% of subcutaneously injected insulin enters the circulation by local absorption across the capillary wall and 50% via the lymphatics

(e) Some insulin preparations become shorter-acting during an acidosis

MTF Question 21

Regarding coaxial breathing systems, which of the following are true?

(a) The use of a coaxial breathing system will allow the use of a lower fresh gas flow (FGF) without re-breathing compared to the non-coaxial equivalent system

(b) The coaxial form of the Mapleson D breathing system is known as the Bain circuit

(c) The diameter of the external breathing hose on a coaxial system is similar to the diameter of the breathing hose in a non-coaxial system

(d) Disconnection of the inner lumen of a Bain circuit may cause a rise in the inspired CO_2 concentration

(e) The Lack circuit is functionally similar to a Mapleson A system

MTF Question 22

Furosemide:

(a) Is not as effective a diuretic as a thiazide in patients with chronic kidney disease

(b) Is more likely to cause deafness in patients with nephrotic syndrome

(c) Reduces both cardiac preload and afterload before causing a diuresis

(d) Potentiates the nephrotoxicity of gentamicin

(e) Causes a diuresis that is enhanced by the co-administration of non-steroidal anti-inflammatory drugs

MTF Question 23

Which of the following statements regarding enzyme induction and inhibition are correct?

(a) Phenytoin increases the metabolism of certain drugs, including tricyclic antidepressants
(b) Induction of an enzyme is caused solely by increased gene expression
(c) Metronidazole enhances the toxicity of ethanol
(d) Aminophylline has an increased duration of action in smokers
(e) Rifampicin enhances the toxicity of ethanol

MTF Question 24

Which of the following are true?

(a) The SI unit of dynamic viscosity is a newton·second/metre
(b) The viscosity of blood is dependent on flow rate
(c) A thixotropic material is a material that becomes less viscous over time when it is agitated or otherwise stressed
(d) The dynamic viscosity of a gas is independent of pressure
(e) The relationship between viscosity and temperature and pressure only holds true for those fluids and gases that exhibit 'Newtonian' properties

MTF Question 25

Which of the following statements are correct with regard to units of measurement?

(a) A tall adult male with a weight of 686 N would not be considered obese
(b) One kilocalorie is equal to 4.2 joules
(c) Pipeline pressure on the anaesthetic machine is equal to 3000 mmHg
(d) Normal body temperature is approximately equal to 97.8 °F
(e) A mean arterial blood pressure of 109 cmH_2O is not compatible with life

MTF Question 26

Regarding a valve block that is attached to a medical gas cylinder:

(a) There is a metal seal between the valve and cylinder that will melt at 70 °C, thus reducing the risk of explosion
(b) It is marked with the tare weight of the cylinder
(c) It is marked with the chemical symbol of the gas contained in the cylinder
(d) It is marked with the name of the gas contained in the cylinder
(e) There is a unique serial number stamped on each valve block

MTF Question 27

Regarding acid–base balance:

(a) Plasma bicarbonate concentration is increased by urinary excretion of hydrogen
(b) Renal filtration of hydrogen ions contributes significantly to the maintenance of a normal plasma pH
(c) The reabsorption of bicarbonate by the renal tubules is dependent on hydrogen excretion
(d) In the collecting tubule, secreted hydrogen will most likely combine with phosphate, not bicarbonate
(e) Bicarbonate is freely filtered at the glomerulus

MTF Question 28

Regarding the functional anatomy of the liver, which of the following are correct?

(a) There are three lobes of the liver
(b) The Couinaud classification describes eight functional segments of the liver
(c) The quadrate lobe is segment 1
(d) Segment 1 is not visible anteriorly
(e) The Bismuth classification divides segment 4 into 4a and 4b

MTF Question 29

Causes of neuropathic pain include:

(a) Carpal tunnel syndrome
(b) Persistent immobility
(c) Shingles
(d) Bipolar depression
(e) Multiple sclerosis

MTF Question 30

The sarcomere is the basic contractile unit of skeletal muscle. Which of the following statements are true?

(a) Myosin filaments make up the A band
(b) The H band is the central area where myosin is not overlapped by actin
(c) The thin filament is composed of two myosin filaments wound together with tropomyosin
(d) The Z line maintains the spatial relationship of the thin filaments
(e) Troponin is composed of three subunits: troponin I, troponin T and troponin C

MTF Question 31

Regarding the use of hypertonic saline to control raised intracranial pressure (ICP):

(a) Patients require regular measurement of serum osmolality for therapeutic monitoring
(b) The high sodium load makes hypertonic saline more of a potential danger to renal function than mannitol
(c) Hypertonic saline should be avoided in hyponatraemic patients
(d) Patients receiving hypertonic saline are more haemodynamically stable than those receiving mannitol
(e) Current evidence would indicate that hypertonic saline produces a longer-lasting fall in ICP than mannitol osmotherapy

MTF Question 32

Regarding the management of chronic obstructive pulmonary disease (COPD):

(a) In the absence of significant contraindications, systemic corticosteroids should be prescribed routinely for all patients with exacerbation of COPD admitted to hospital
(b) Mucolytics such as carbocisteine have no place in the management of stable COPD
(c) More than 15 hours of oxygen a day when on long-term oxygen therapy (LTOT) is undesirable, as outcome deteriorates because of injury by free radicals
(d) LTOT improves quality of life but does not prolong survival

Paper 1

(e) A patient with an infective exacerbation of COPD should only be given a maximum FiO$_2$ of 0.3 because of the risk of removing hypoxic drive

MTF Question 33

Regarding the pharmacological management of hypertension:

(a) An angiotensin-converting enzyme (ACE) inhibitor would be better than a thiazide diuretic as a first-line drug in a 50-year-old female Caucasian patient with hypertension
(b) A trial of single agent use should be assessed at 4 weeks
(c) Management should target lowering blood pressure to below 140/90 mmHg
(d) Severe hypertension (>180/110 mmHg) usually requires a different group of drugs to the standard hypertension treatment plan
(e) Spironolactone would be the best diuretic to add to management of a patient uncontrolled on triple therapy

MTF Question 34

Regarding antigen presentation, which of the following statements are correct?

(a) Macrophages are capable of presenting foreign particles to B lymphocytes
(b) Dendrites, present on antigen-presenting cells, improve interaction with T cells
(c) T-cell receptors will recognise antigens presented via the human leucocyte antigen but not the major histocompatibility complex
(d) Antigen-presenting cells include epithelial cells
(e) Activation of T helper cells stimulates further proliferation of human leucocyte antigen molecules on macrophages

MTF Question 35

With regard to the use of endotracheal tubes in children, which of the following statements are true?

(a) The glottis is the narrowest part of the airway in children
(b) According to Cole's formula the correct size for a 4-year-old would be 5.0 mm internal diameter
(c) Nasal endotracheal tubes should be avoided in children under 8 years
(d) Uncuffed tubes are not suitable for rapid sequence induction
(e) According to Cole's formula the correct size for a 6-year-old would be 6.5 mm internal diameter

MTF Question 36

Regarding vitamin K:

(a) It is used as prophylaxis against haemolytic disease of the newborn
(b) The body carries no significant stores of vitamin K
(c) It is so named because it was discovered after vitamin J (biotin)
(d) It is required for the activation of some anticoagulant factors
(e) Synthetic oral vitamin K should not be administered to neonates

MTF Question 37

Which of the following statements about propofol are true?

(a) Propofol is contraindicated in patients with an allergy to eggs

(b) Excitatory movements seen on induction with propofol are due to epileptiform EEG activity
(c) Propofol is 75% protein-bound in plasma
(d) Propofol causes more cardiovascular changes than thiopental when used in equi-analgesic doses
(e) Pain on injection of propofol can be reduced by injecting into a fast-flowing intravenous drip

MTF Question 38

Which of the following statements correctly describe the principles of impedance?

(a) The unit of impedance is the same as that of resistance
(b) Impedance is given the symbol Ω
(c) Skin impedance is lower when the skin is moist
(d) Defibrillation may be more effective during inspiration than expiration
(e) Impedance is inversely proportional to current frequency

MTF Question 39

Regarding sedation in children and young adults:

(a) Fasting is not required for minimal sedation
(b) Intravenous propofol, with or without fentanyl or intravenous ketamine, is recommended for deep sedation for painful procedures
(c) Intravenous midazolam with fentanyl is recommended for upper gastrointestinal endoscopy
(d) Opioids are not recommended for non-painful procedures
(e) Chloral hydrate has no place in the sedation of children

MTF Question 40

Draw-over vaporisers:

(a) Are driven by downstream negative pressure
(b) Have a high resistance to flow
(c) Are often used 'in the field' because of their portability
(d) Require an external cylinder gas supply
(e) Are positioned inside the breathing system

MTF Question 41

The Tec Mk 6 vaporiser:

(a) Is an example of a plenum vaporiser
(b) Has a chamber operating temperature of 29 °C
(c) Is made of copper
(d) Has a warm-up time of 30 seconds
(e) Requires an external power supply

MTF Question 42

Which of the following statements about drug uptake are true?

(a) Hepatic first-pass metabolism of propranolol is influenced by the degree of protein binding

(b) Rectal administration of drugs improves absorption compared to oral administration

(c) Vecuronium is ionised in the stomach and largely absorbed in the small intestine

(d) Where hepatic metabolic capacity for a drug is high, first-pass metabolism is dependent on hepatic blood flow

(e) Nasal administration has the advantage of rapid onset of action

MTF Question 43

Which of the following statements correctly describes the structure of epidural equipment?

(a) The bevel of the epidural needle is angled at 30° to the shaft
(b) The bevel of the Tuohy needle is known as a Crawford point
(c) The paediatric Tuohy needle has markings in 0.5 cm increments
(d) The epidural catheter is made of PTFE
(e) Fluid does not leave through the tip of the epidural catheter; it only exits through side ports

MTF Question 44

Which of the following are true regarding the adjustable pressure-limiting (APL) valve?

(a) The APL valve allows positive-pressure ventilation when completely unscrewed
(b) During periods of high flow (e.g. at peak inspiration), it is possible to entrain room air through the APL valve during spontaneous respiration
(c) Modern APL valves incorporate a secondary overpressure relief valve, which prevents the circuit pressure rising above 60 cmH_2O
(d) The overpressure relief valve is redundant in modern breathing circuits, as the distensible reservoir bag prevents excessive pressure rises
(e) The APL valve will produce positive end-expiratory pressure (PEEP)

MTF Question 45

Iron absorption:

(a) Primarily occurs in the terminal ileum
(b) Is independent of total body stores
(c) Is extremely efficient
(d) Occurs via active transport
(e) Binds apoferritin once inside intestinal cells

MTF Question 46

Regarding the measurement of peak expiratory flow rate:

(a) Results depend on patient effort
(b) It may be measured with a pneumotachograph
(c) It is the maximal rate of airflow during passive expiration
(d) Normal values in females are 350–600 mL/min
(e) Normal values in males are 450–700 L/min

MTF Question 47

In the perioperative management of a patient having surgery for carcinoid syndrome:

(a) Thiopental would be a good choice of induction agent
(b) Morphine would be a good choice of narcotic analgesic

(c) Intraoperative hypotension may be improved by the administration of octreotide

(d) Regional anaestheisa avoids most of the major complications caused by general anaesthesia

(e) Ondansetron is the agent of choice to prevent postoperative nausea and vomiting

MTF Question 48

Regarding thyroid hormone secretion and thyroid-stimulating hormone (TSH):

(a) TSH increases the uptake of thyroid hormones by thyroglobulin

(b) Thyroxine-binding globulin (TBG) has the greatest capacity to bind thyroxine compared with other plasma proteins

(c) Reduced protein binding results in increased free hormone

(d) Cold increases circulating TSH levels

(e) Glucocorticoids stimulate TSH secretion

MTF Question 49

Regarding sickle cell disease, which of the following statements are true?

(a) Sickle cell disease is due to a single DNA base change on the β-globin chain, rendering the molecule more hydrophilic

(b) The affinity of dissolved sickle haemoglobin for oxygen is the same as that of normal haemoglobin

(c) The degree of precipitation of sickle haemoglobin is dependent on the concentration of deoxygenated haemoglobin.

(d) A patient with sickle cell disease may also have normal haemoglobin A

(e) Sickle haemoglobin precipitates at a PO_2 of 3–4 kPa

MTF Question 50

Which of the following are true regarding the measurement of gas and vapour concentrations?

(a) The presence of water vapour in a sample will increase the concentration of other gases

(b) Saturated vapour pressure is needed to correct for water vapour

(c) Barometric pressure is needed to correct for water vapour

(d) Water vapour can be removed by silica gel

(e) Water vapour is removed by modern gas analysers

MTF Question 51

Regarding suxamethonium:

(a) It is a dicholine ester of succinic acid

(b) When presented as the bromide salt it is supplied as a powder and needs to be dissolved in sterile water before use

(c) It is made up of two molecules of acetylcholine (ACh) joined via their hydroxyl groups

(d) It can be presented as the fluoride salt

(e) When presented as the chloride salt it is supplied as a 100 mg/mL solution

MTF Question 52

Regarding the bispectral index (BIS) value scale, which of the following are true?

(a) A value of 80 represents an awake patient

(b) A value of 40–60 is recommended for general anaesthesia

(c) Patient temperature has no effect on the BIS value
(d) Cerebral ischaemia reduces the BIS value
(e) A value of zero indicates a flatline EEG

MTF Question 53

Regarding insulin and the insulin receptor:

(a) Insulin has a tertiary protein structure
(b) Insulin is produced from preproinsulin in the endoplasmic reticulum
(c) The insulin receptor has two α and two β subunits.
(d) Receptor binding results in production of cell membrane transporters
(e) The insulin receptor activates adenylyl cyclase via a second-messenger system

MTF Question 54

Regarding the use of antidepressants for pain, which of the following statements are true?

(a) The dose of amitriptyline to treat neuropathic pain is higher than the dose required to treat depression
(b) The onset of analgesic action is slower than the onset of antidepressant action
(c) Amitriptyline is licensed for use in neuropathic pain
(d) Nortriptyline is less sedative than amitriptyline
(e) Selective serotonin reuptake inhibitors are more effective than the tricyclic antidepressants in treating pain

MTF Question 55

Which of the following statements regarding circle systems are true?

(a) Calcium hydroxide is found in soda lime and is re-formed during the reaction with carbon dioxide
(b) Low-flow anaesthesia with a circle system is safe in patients who are intoxicated
(c) A 500 g canister of soda lime can absorb > 120 L of carbon dioxide gas
(d) Prolonged low-flow anaesthesia with sevoflurane produces proteinuria, glycosuria and enzymuria, which can be detrimental to patients with pre-existing biochemical evidence of renal dysfunction
(e) During low-flow anaesthesia, carboxyhaemoglobin levels may approach 3–4%

MTF Question 56

Regarding the anatomy of the circle of Willis:

(a) One-third of the blood supply is from internal carotid arteries
(b) The anterior cerebral artery supplies the superior and medial parts of the cerebral hemispheres
(c) The middle communicating artery joins the internal carotid artery and posterior cerebral artery
(d) The middle cerebral artery supplies the lateral aspect of the cerebral hemispheres
(e) The superior cerebellar artery is a branch of the posterior inferior cerebellar artery

MTF Question 57

Which of the following statements regarding inflammatory mediators are correct?

(a) Leukotrienes cause vasodilation
(b) The kinin system mediates increased capillary permeability

(c) Tumour necrosis factor is a cytokine produced mainly by granulocytes
(d) Histamine is produced by basophils
(e) Chemokines, such as interleukin 8, are involved in chemotaxis

MTF Question 58

Regarding olfactory receptors:

(a) Olfactory receptors project through the cribiform plate in the sphenoid bone
(b) Adjacent basal cells produce mucus
(c) Chemoreceptors are directly triggered by odiferous chemicals in the airflow
(d) Sustenacular cells continually produce more olfactory receptors
(e) Olfactory receptors have a half-life of one month

MTF Question 59

The following physiological changes may be seen when commencing a noradrenaline infusion at 12 µg/minute:

(a) Increased insulin secretion
(b) Coronary vasodilation
(c) Even with no change in perfusion pressure, renal blood flow will increase
(d) Miosis
(e) Pregnant uterine muscle relaxation

MTF Question 60

The components of dietary lipids have different functions. Which of the following are true regarding the components of dietary lipid?

(a) Fatty acids are the body's main form of stored energy
(b) Fatty acid chains are stored in triglycerides
(c) Triglycerides are transported free in the plasma
(d) Lipoproteins have specific roles for different tissue targets
(e) Phospholipids form structural components of cell membranes

SBA Question 61

Consider a hypothetical situation in which the following gases or vapours are stored separately in cylinders in a hot operating theatre (the thermometer reads 35 °C). Which one of the following would NOT contain gas alone, irrespective of the pressure within the cylinder?

(a) Oxygen
(b) Nitrogen
(c) Nitrous oxide
(d) Carbon dioxide
(e) Air

(SBA Question 62

You are asked to provide anaesthesia for a pregnant woman undergoing emergency appendicectomy. Of the following drugs administered to the woman, which is the least likely to accumulate in the fetus?

(a) Bupivacaine
(b) Pethidine

(c) Thiopental
(d) Diamorphine
(e) Diazepam

SBA Question 63

A patient on the intensive care unit is being ventilated in a volume-controlled mode with an FiO_2 of 0.6. Arterial blood gas analysis reveals a PaO_2 of 7.5 kPa and a $PaCO_2$ of 4.7 kPa. Which ONE of the following is the best intervention aimed at increasing the PaO_2?

(a) Increase the FiO_2
(b) Increase the tidal volume
(c) Increase the frequency
(d) Increase the inspiratory time
(e) Increase the expiratory time

SBA Question 64

Regarding the management of acute myocardial infarction presenting with ischaemic symptoms and persistent ST elevation, which ONE of the following would be an absolute contraindication to fibrinolytic therapy?

(a) Previous fibrinolysis 5 months ago
(b) Resuscitated cardiac arrest within the last hour
(c) Diabetic retinopathy
(d) Ischaemic stroke 2 months ago
(e) Pregnant at 36 weeks gestation

SBA Question 65

A new drug is being tested. Its onset of action depends on the rate of diffusion across the cell membrane. The following factors increase the rate of diffusion of a substance across a biological membrane, EXCEPT which one?

(a) Decreased molecular weight
(b) Increased concentration gradient
(c) Decreased solubility of a gas
(d) Increased lipid solubility
(e) For a weakly acidic substance, a low environmental pH

SBA Question 66

A hormone is produced in the cytoplasm of an endocrine cell and is then stored in granules within the cytoplasm. On release from the cell it is carried in the bloodstream to a target cell, where it crosses the cell membrane and binds directly to the nucleus, increasing cell gene transcription. Which hormone is best described in these terms?

(a) Adrenaline
(b) Thyroxine
(c) Aldosterone
(d) Thyroid-stimulating hormone
(e) Growth hormone

SBA Question 67

A 52-year-old male with no comorbidities is undergoing a right hemicolectomy for bowel carcinoma. His pulse is 70 beats/min, his blood pressure is 90/55 mmHg. An oesophageal Doppler displays the following variables: cardiac output 4.2 L/min, stroke volume 43 mL, flow time corrected (FTc) 300, peak velocity (PV) 55 cm/second. Which ONE of the following would be the best intervention?

(a) Start an infusion of dopexamine
(b) Start an infusion of dobutamine
(c) Give a 200 mL fluid challenge
(d) Start an infusion of noradrenaline
(e) Give a 500 mL fluid challenge

SBA Question 68

An adult patient in the recovery room develops a narrow-complex AV nodal re-entry tachycardia. The patient has an acceptable blood pressure and no signs of myocardial ischaemia or heart failure. Vagal manoeuvres followed by a rapid 6 mg bolus of intravenous adenosine have failed to change the rhythm. Which of the following would represent the best practice for immediate ongoing management?

(a) Anaesthetise and perform DC cardioversion
(b) Administer 12 mg of intravenous adenosine
(c) Administer 300 mg of intravenous amiodarone
(d) Administer 2.5 mg of intravenous verapamil
(e) Administer 5 mg of intravenous metoprolol

SBA Question 69

An elderly man is admitted into the medical admission unit with a sudden deterioration in vision. Examination of the visual fields reveals loss of vision in only the right side of the visual field in both eyes (right homonymous hemianopia). Where in the visual pathway is the lesion?

(a) Right optic nerve
(b) Left optic nerve
(c) Optic chiasm
(d) Right optic radiation
(e) Left optic radiation

SBA Question 70

You are discussing with a colleague anatomical sites used to measure core temperature in a patient under anaesthesia. Which of your colleague's following statements regarding temperature measurement is NOT correct?

(a) The tympanic membrane is a useful site from which to sample temperature, as it closely correlates with hypothalamic temperature and has a rapid response time
(b) Temperature sampled from the upper third of the oesophagus accurately reflects core body temperature
(c) Bladder temperature measurement is more accurate at high urine flow rates than low urine flow rates
(d) Rectal temperature is usually 0.5–1 °C higher than core body temperature
(e) Core body temperature is measured accurately and continuously from the pulmonary artery

SBA Question 71

You have been training hard for over a year in preparation for an 'Ironman' triathlon race in Switzerland in the summer. You would expect all of the following changes to occur with this endurance training, EXCEPT which one?

(a) Significant increase in the resting stroke volume as well as maximal exercise stroke volume
(b) Increased resting oxygen uptake, from 0.3 L/min to 0.5 L/min
(c) Increased maximum oxygen uptake, from 2.8 L/min to 5.2 L/min
(d) Hypertrophy of the heart, which is similar to the effects of hypertension
(e) Delayed exercise-related rise in lactate

SBA Question 72

Whilst in theatre with an anaesthetised, intubated and ventilated patient, you notice interference on your ECG trace. What would be the most likely explanation for this interference?

(a) The patient must be in contact with live electrical equipment
(b) Direct current can pass from a theatre lamp
(c) Electrons can flow directly across an air gap
(d) The patient can behave like one plate of a capacitor
(e) The patient is moving

SBA Question 73

A 80-year-old woman is treated for New York Heart Association (NYHA) class II heart failure. On a routine visit to her GP she is noted to have palpable pitting oedema to her mid calf. Which of the following best describes the mechanism by which this is occurring?

(a) Increased proximal capillary hydrostatic pressure
(b) Increased distal capillary hydrostatic pressure
(c) Decreased proximal capillary hydrostatic pressure
(d) Decreased distal capillary hydrostatic pressure
(e) Increased interstitial hydrostatic pressure

SBA Question 74

Which of the following is the most accurate description of the flow in a Rotameter?

(a) It demonstrates turbulent flow throughout
(b) It demonstrates laminar flow throughout
(c) It demonstrates variable pressure throughout
(d) For any given flow rate setting, the Reynolds number increases towards the top of the Rotameter
(e) Calibration depends on both density and viscosity

SBA Question 75

An abnormal Valsalva response may be detected when assessing patients with a number of pathological conditions such as diabetic, peripheral neuropathy. Which of the following statements about abnormal Valsalva responses is INCORRECT?

(a) Autonomic dysfunction causes the blood pressure to fall and remain low until phase III
(b) A square-wave response may be seen in hypovolaemic patients
(c) No change in heart rate is observed in patients with autonomic dysfunction
(d) The blood pressure rises but does not fall in patients with cardiac tamponade
(e) Abnormal Valsalva can be demonstrated after sympathectomy

SBA Question 76

A patient with chronic obstructive pulmonary disease presents for assessment for long-term oxygen therapy (LTOT) and is found to have a compensated respiratory acidosis. Which of the following sets of arterial blood gases best demonstrates compensated respiratory acidosis?

(a) pH $= 7.30$, $PCO_2 = 7.2$ kPa, $PO_2 = 9.5$ kPa, $HCO_3^- = 25$ mmol/L
(b) pH $= 7.36$, $PCO_2 = 8.5$ kPa, $PO_2 = 7.5$ kPa, $HCO_3^- = 43$ mmol/L
(c) pH $= 7.24$, $PCO_2 = 10.1$ kPa, $PO_2 = 7.0$ kPa, $HCO_3^- = 27$ mmol/L
(d) pH $= 7.24$, $PCO_2 = 3.5$ kPa, $PO_2 = 8.5$ kPa, $HCO_3^- = 18$ mmol/L
(e) pH $= 7.20$, $PCO_2 = 6.2$ kPa, $PO_2 = 9.0$ kPa, $HCO_3^- = 15$ mmol/L

SBA Question 77

Consider anaesthetising 100 identical patients who were all 50-year-old non-smokers with a strong previous history of postoperative nausea and vomiting (PONV) scheduled for a total abdominal hysterectomy. You are likely to use an opioid for intraoperative and postoperative analgesia. How many of the 100 would be prevented from suffering PONV by the intraoperative administration of 4 mg intravenous ondansetron?

(a) 5
(b) 10
(c) 20
(d) 50
(e) 80

SBA Question 78

Which of the following statements regarding humoral mechanisms involved in controlling haemorrhage is INCORRECT?

(a) Circulating catecholamines increase
(b) Atrial natriuretic peptide (ANP) levels increase
(c) Vasopressin release is mediated via the Gauer–Henry reflex
(d) Stimulation of the adrenal cortex promotes release of aldosterone
(e) Circulating levels of enkephalins increase

SBA Question 79

Capnography is part of the AAGBI minimal monitoring requirements for general anaesthesia. Regarding capnography, which of following is the LEAST correct?

(a) Capnography is based on the principle that gases with two or more different atoms in the molecule will absorb infrared radiation
(b) The particular frequency of infrared radiation is selected by first passing it through a crystal window
(c) A reference cell increases accuracy of the system
(d) The use of infrared radiation with a wavelength of 4.28 μm for the analysis of carbon dioxide should reduce interference from the presence of nitrous oxide
(e) In the sidestream capnograph, a sample is drawn at about 150 mL/min

SBA Question 80

When a standard dose of lidocaine without vasoconstrictor is injected into various different sites around the body, care is taken to avoid intravascular injection and peak plasma levels of lidocaine are measured after injection. Which ONE of the following ranks the various sites correctly in terms of plasma concentration of lidocaine? The site producing the highest plasma concentration is ranked first.

(a) Brachial plexus, epidural, intercostal, caudal
(b) Caudal, brachial plexus, intercostal, epidural
(c) Epidural, intercostal, brachial plexus, caudal
(d) Epidural, caudal, brachial plexus, intercostal
(e) Intercostal, caudal, epidural, brachial plexus

SBA Question 81

A farmer slips and falls in a remote field during a hot summer. He has nothing to eat and his only drink is whisky from a hip flask. He is not found for 3 days. On admission to hospital he is peripherally cold, with a heart rate of 110 beats/min and a blood pressure of 85/40 mmHg. Which of the following is the most potent stimulus for antidiuretic hormone release?

Answers:
(a) Stimulation of central osmoreceptors
(b) Stimulation of aortic arch baroreceptors
(c) Ingestion of alcohol
(d) Pain
(e) Stress

SBA Question 82

An adult patient distressed by shivering in the postoperative period would be most effectively treated with which ONE of the following?

(a) Pethidine 25 mg
(b) Doxapram 100 mg
(c) Clonidine 150 µg
(d) Ketanserin 10 mg
(e) Alfentanil 250 µg

SBA Question 83

A group of doctors from your hospital have recently returned from a charity trip climbing Mount Everest. They are relieved to be home as they said that they couldn't have a good cup of tea on the mountain. Which of these responses would best explain why?

(a) The boiling point of water is 373.15 kelvin
(b) The boiling point is the temperature of a substance at which its saturated vapour pressure equals external atmospheric pressure
(c) A gas is a substance at a temperature above its critical temperature
(d) Boiling point increases with increasing pressure
(e) The saturated vapour pressure of a substance increases with increasing temperature

SBA Question 84

It is important to understand the physiological control of normal respiration. Considering a normal, unstressed, spontaneously respiring patient, which ONE of the following is considered to be most the important factor in regulating resting ventilation?

(a) The effect of arterial oxygen tension at the central chemoreceptors
(b) Changes in cerebrospinal fluid pH at the central chemoreceptors
(c) The effect of arterial CO_2 tension at the peripheral chemoreceptors
(d) Changes in plasma pH at peripheral chemoreceptors
(e) The effect of arterial oxygen tension at the peripheral chemoreceptors

SBA Question 85

Minimum inhibitory concentration (MIC) may be used in the laboratory assessment of the efficacy of a particular antibiotic in the treatment of a particular organism. Which ONE of the following is the best definition of MIC?

(a) MIC is the average plasma concentration caused by administering the lowest scheduled dose of an antibiotic
(b) MIC is the lowest concentration of antibiotic required to kill 50% of bacterial colonies on a laboratory culture plate within 24 hours at standard temperature
(c) MIC is the optimal concentration targeted for trough readings during therapeutic monitoring
(d) MIC is the lowest concentration of an antimicrobial that will inhibit the visible growth of a microorganism after overnight incubation
(e) MIC is the minimum antibiotic concentration in the plasma of adult humans required to cause a reduction in yield from blood cultures

SBA Question 86

A 68-year-old female is about to have an emergency laparotomy for suspected perforated colonic diverticulum. She looks unwell. She chronically has an eGFR of 33 mL/min/1.73 m^2 and weighs 80 kg. Which ONE of the following intravenous antibiotic regimens would you consider to be best in these circumstances?

(a) Cefuroxime 1.5 g and metronidazole 500 mg
(b) Gentamicin 240 mg and teicoplanin 800 mg
(c) Vancomycin 1 g and gentamicin 160 mg
(d) Tazocin 3.375 g
(e) Gentamicin 160 mg, benzylpenicillin 1.8 g and metronidazole 500 mg

SBA Question 87

Ambulance control warns you that you are expecting a major incident in to your emergency department following exposure of eight people to a large dose of organophosphate (OP) insecticide. The patients have been decontaminated at the scene but are symptomatic of OP toxicity. Given the choice of a range of drug packs, which ONE would you choose?

(a) Pack A contains diazepam, atropine, pralidoxime and ecothiopate
(b) Pack B contains diazepam, atropine, suxamethonium and ecothiopate
(c) Pack C contains diazepam, pralidoxime, suxamethonium and neostigmine
(d) Pack D contains atropine, pralidoxime, suxamethonium and neostigmine
(e) Pack E contains atropine, pralidoxime neostigmine and ecothiopate

SBA Question 88

A patient with factor V Leiden deficiency presents with pleuritic pain and shortness of breath. Which ONE of the following tests would be most appropriate to investigate this patient for a pulmonary embolus?

(a) Radioisotope scanning using xenon and technetium
(b) Spirometry
(c) Analysis of single-breath nitrogen washout
(d) Radioisotope scanning using xenon and strontium
(e) Lung function tests

SBA Question 89

The circulation of blood in the fetus differs from the adult circulation, and circulating blood has reduced oxygen saturations. In order of descending magnitude, order the following vessels according to their normal fetal saturations: umbilical artery (UA); umbilical vein (UV); superior vena cava (SVC); inferior vena cava (IVC); ductus venosus (DV); ductus arteriosus (DA).

(a) UA, DV, IVC, UV, DA, SVC
(b) UV, DV, IVC, DA, UA, SVC
(c) UV, IVC, DV, UA, DA, SVC
(d) UA, DV, IVC, SVC, DA, UV
(e) UV, DV, IVC, SVC, DA, UA

SBA Question 90

A 38-year-old man smokes 40 cigarettes a day. An arterial blood gas taken in air shows him to have a PaO_2 of 95 mmHg, a $PaCO_2$ of 39 mmHg, a carboxyhaemoglobin (COHb) concentration of 6% and Hb of 13.5. Approximately where on the oxyhaemoglobin dissociation curve will his P_{50} be?

(a) 5.3
(b) 4.1
(c) 3.8
(d) 3.5
(e) 2.9

Paper 2

MTF Question 1

When prescribing in the postoperative period:

(a) Chronic pain analgesia should be stopped because of the risk of toxicity and interactions with acute pain analgesia
(b) Supplementary analgesia beyond codeine should be prescribed, as the efficacy of codeine varies hugely from individual to individual
(c) An antiemetic should be prescribed to all patients who have had a general anaesthetic
(d) A laxative such as lactulose should be prescribed to all elderly patients who have been prescribed postoperative opioids
(e) Unless contraindicated, paracetamol should be prescribed 'as required' for all patients

MTF Question 2

With regard to the environmental control of the operating theatre, which of the following statements correctly describe passive scavenging systems?

(a) 33 mm tubing is used in the transfer system
(b) Volatile anaesthetic agents can be recirculated, saving money through conservation of use
(c) The use of nitrous oxide may reduce the efficiency of the system
(d) Atmospheric conditions may affect the cardiopulmonary status of the patient through the use of a passive scavenging system
(e) Atmospheric pollution is greater than with the active scavenging system

MTF Question 3

Which of the following statements about ion channels are correct?

(a) Voltage-gated ion channels can be either open or closed
(b) The binding site of a ligand-gated ion channel is usually in the extracellular domain
(c) The β_2-adrenoreceptor is an example of a ligand-gated ion channel
(d) The duration of opening of voltage-gated channels is purely controlled by the membrane potential of the cell
(e) The NMDA glutamate receptor exhibits both voltage-gated and ligand-gated activation

MTF Question 4

Regarding the parasympathetic nervous system:

(a) Cranial nerves III, VII, VIII and X carry parasympathetic afferent fibres to the pupil and salivary glands
(b) Sacral outflow originates from the 2nd, 3rd and 4th sacral segments of the spinal cord
(c) The vagus nerve innervates the ureter
(d) Bronchial muscle constriction is mediated via thoracic fibres
(e) Sacral fibres innervate the distal colon, rectum, bladder and reproductive organs

MTF Question 5

Regarding the cardiovascular changes associated with pregnancy:

(a) Significant cardiovascular changes can be observed by week 8 gestation
(b) Heart rate increases most in the third trimester
(c) Aortocaval compression typically becomes a problem around 16 weeks
(d) A 10–15 mmHg rise in mean arterial pressure is typical
(e) Cardiac output returns to pre-pregnancy levels by 48 hours postpartum

MTF Question 6

Regarding vomiting centre afferents:

(a) The mechano- and chemoreceptors in the gastrointestinal tract are both vagal nerve afferents
(b) The vomiting centre is a discrete area of reticular formation in the medulla
(c) The vomiting centre receives afferent fibres from cranial nerves V, VII, IX, X and XII
(d) Cranial nerve X is the predominant afferent input from the heart
(e) Raised intracranial pressure on the third ventricle stimulates vomiting

(MTF Question 7

Regarding the use of epidural analgesia with low-dose bupivacaine and fentanyl in labour:

(a) Epidural analgesia produces a reduced Apgar score at 1 minute but not at 5 minutes
(b) Women receiving an epidural are more likely to have a forceps or vacuum delivery
(c) Epidural analgesia increases the risk of a caesarean section
(d) The siting of an epidural increases the likelihood of long-term postpartum backache
(e) It is not uncommon for women receiving an epidural to have a significant rise in body temperature

MTF Question 8

Which of the following will reduce the power of statistical analysis?

(a) Increasing the sample size
(b) Decreasing the significance level
(c) Increasing the probability of a type two (beta) error
(d) Increasing the probability of a type one (alpha) error
(e) Decreasing the magnitude of the effect of the treatment intervention

MTF Question 9

Which of the following statements about the pharmacological effects of renal failure are correct?

(a) Vecuronium should be avoided in patients with acute kidney injury
(b) Patients with renal failure may require a higher loading dose of a drug in order to achieve a therapeutic plasma concentration
(c) Dose reductions can be calculated by multiplying the usual dose by the ratio of the patient's creatinine clearance and a normal creatinine clearance
(d) The targeted plasma concentration of a drug will be the same in renal failure as in a healthy patient
(e) Renal failure causes accumulation of propofol and prolongs the effect of propofol infusion

MTF Question 10

Regarding the mechanism of action of non-steroidal anti-inflammatory drugs (NSAIDs):

(a) They inhibit the enzymes cyclooxygenase and lipoxygenase in the metabolism of arachidonic acid
(b) Their antipyretic activity is brought about via reduced production of PGE_2
(c) Increased levels of leukotrienes are as a result of increased activity of lipoxygenase
(d) Production of phospholipase A_2 is reduced
(e) Platelet production of prostacyclin is inhibited

MTF Question 11

Which of the following statements regarding catecholamine synthesis and metabolism are correct?

(a) Tyrosine is converted from phenylalanine by decarboxylation
(b) Dopamine is the first catecholamine formed through the synthetic pathway
(c) Tyrosine hydroxylase facilitates the rate-limiting step
(d) Noradrenaline is converted to adrenaline by the enzyme catechol-O-methyltransferase
(e) Monoamine oxidase is involved in the metabolism of catecholamines

MTF Question 12

The P_{50}:
(a) Is the arterial oxygen tension at which haemoglobin saturation is 50%
(b) Moves to the right according to the Bohr effect
(c) Is typically less than 3.5 kPa in the presence of carbon monoxide poisoning
(d) Represents the haemoglobin saturation when arterial oxygen tension is 50 mmHg
(e) Shifts to the left in fetal blood

MTF Question 13

Regarding the cardiac cycle in a healthy adult:

(a) In a healthy heart coronary perfusion to both ventricles occurs primarily during diastole
(b) During systole, the aortic valve opens at approximately 120 mmHg, reflecting the systolic blood pressure
(c) The dicrotic notch marks the end of systole
(d) The right ventricle reaches maximum pressures of 25 mmHg during systole
(e) During systole, the pressure gradient between left ventricle and aorta is less than 5 mmHg

MTF Question 14

Which of the following are true regarding opioid receptors?

(a) All opioid receptors are ionotropic
(b) All opioid receptors are metabotropic
(c) The opioid receptors are coupled to Gs proteins
(d) There are four classical opioid receptors
(e) Ketocyclazacine is an antagonist at all endogenous opioid receptors

MTF Question 15

Which of the following statements regarding the control of blood volume are correct?

(a) Low-pressure baroreceptors are located in the carotid sinus
(b) The juxtaglomerular apparatus releases angiotensinogen in response to sympathetic activity
(c) The arterial baroreceptor reflex transmits signals to higher centres via the glossopharyngeal nerve
(d) The thirst sensation is partially mediated by antidiuretic hormone
(e) Long-term control includes redistribution of blood from reservoirs

MTF Question 16

Which of the following combinations correctly describes a neurotransmitter (stated first) matched with the receptor at which it is an agonist (stated second)?

(a) α-Amino-3-hydroxy-5-methyl-4-isoxazole-propionate (AMPA) and N-methyl-D-aspartate (NMDA)
(b) Substance P and neurokinin 1
(c) Glutamate and γ-aminobutyric acid A ($GABA_A$)
(d) Glycine and NMDA
(e) Kainate and glutamate

MTF Question 17

Which of the following statements concerning osmolality are true?

(a) Plasma osmolality ranges from 280 to 295 mOsm/L
(b) Osmolality of body fluid is usually higher than its osmolarity
(c) Antidiuretic hormone is secreted in response to a drop in osmolality
(d) Osmolality is maintained constant throughout the body compartments
(e) Osmolality is regulated by osmoreceptors located in the brainstem

MTF Question 18

Regarding non-depolarising neuromuscular blocking agents:

(a) The neuromuscular block is antagonised by administration of anticholinesterases
(b) Fade to a 1 Hz stimulus is present when there is partial neuromuscular block
(c) The diaphragm is paralysed at lower doses than the adductor policis muscle
(d) Post-tetanic potentiation is seen when there is partial neuromuscular block
(e) Monitoring of the adductor policis muscle is more accurate at reflecting the degree of laryngeal muscle blockade than the orbicularis oculi muscle

MTF Question 19

Regarding starvation:

(a) Glycogen reserves are depleted in less than 24 hours
(b) In early starvation, gluconeogenesis is the main process for glucose production
(c) Protein metabolism leads to an accumulation of acetyl-CoA and the subsequent formation of ketone bodies
(d) As starvation is prolonged, protein breakdown steadily increases
(e) An increase in plasma adrenaline levels results in an increase in plasma fatty acids

MTF Question 20

Regarding topical anaesthetic creams for venepuncture:

(a) EMLA is a eutectic mixture, which in this context means a mixture of substances that have a lower melting point than either of the original substances
(b) Typically, EMLA causes skin blanching
(c) EMLA and Ametop should be stored in a refrigerator below 8 °C
(d) EMLA ideally requires 30 minutes to be fully effective
(e) Lidocaine 4% cream in a liposome base produces minimal skin discolouration and is effective within 30 minutes

MTF Question 21

The medical gases used in anaesthetic practice include medical air, xenon and Heliox. Which of the following statements are true?

(a) Medical air is supplied to anaesthetic machines at a pressure of 7 bar
(b) Medical air is stored in cylinders with black bodies and black and white chequered shoulders at a pressure of 13 700 kPa
(c) Heliox (oxygen/helium mixture) has a lower density than oxygen and therefore is useful in conditions where flow is likely to be laminar
(d) Xenon has a low blood/gas partition coefficient and therefore offers rapid induction of anaesthesia
(e) Xenon is a more potent anaesthetic agent than nitrous oxide

MTF Question 22

Which of the following statements regarding the measurement of flow are correct?

(a) A Rotameter is a flowmeter
(b) The flutes on the bobbin or ridges on the ball of a flowmeter are required to ensure the gas passing it is turbulent in nature
(c) The Fick principle is used to calculate flow
(d) A Venturi accurately measures the flow of gas passing through it
(e) The Wright respirometer may produce inaccurate values if the flow through it is turbulent

MTF Question 23

Which of the following statements regarding the gas laws are true?

(a) Boyle's law is used clinically when assessing the gas contents of an oxygen cylinder
(b) There are 6.022×10^{23} atoms of carbon in 0.012 kg of carbon-12, and this number is used in some gas calculations

(c) The third perfect gas law explains why an oxygen cylinder should not be exposed to extremes of heat

(d) A patient with a pneumothorax boards a commercial aeroplane, and suffers a cardiac arrest when the plane ascends to 32 000 feet – Charles' law explains this phenomenon

(e) At 273.15 K and 101.325 kPa, 1 mol of carbon dioxide gas will occupy 22.4 L. The same is true of 1 mol of argon gas.

MTF Question 24

Which of the following statements about nitrous oxide are true?

(a) Nitrous oxide directly activates opioid receptors
(b) Nitrous oxide oxidises the cobalt ion in vitamin B_{12}
(c) Nitrous oxide should be avoided in the first trimester of pregnancy
(d) Nitrous oxide inhibits glutaminergic transmission at NMDA receptors
(e) Nitrous oxide has a direct myocardial depressant action

MTF Question 25

Regarding anticonvulsants:

(a) They act by either reducing cell membrane ion permeability, enhancing γ-aminobutyric acid receptor activity or inhibiting glutamate receptors
(b) Dosing should vary during the month in the management of catamenial epilepsy
(c) Given in pregnancy they may necessitate oral vitamin K and folic acid supplementation
(d) Carbamazepine is a first-line drug for absence seizures
(e) If a drug needs to be withdrawn rapidly because of toxicity, the patient should be immediately loaded with an alternative anticonvulsant

MTF Question 26

Which of the following statements are correct regarding tests of coagulation?

(a) A prolonged prothrombin time (PT) can be caused by heparin therapy
(b) A prolonged activated partial thromboplastin time (aPTT) may be due to hypofibrinogenaemia
(c) Haemophilia prolongs both PT and aPTT
(d) Thrombin time tests the conversion of prothrombin to thrombin
(e) Von Willebrand's disease affects the PT but not the aPTT

MTF Question 27

Which of the following statements regarding hysteresis are true?

(a) Hysteresis of a monitoring device refers to the ability of the device to respond in both a positive and a negative direction
(b) Hysteresis is a common problem among medical monitoring devices
(c) Hysteresis in a monitoring device is a time-dependent problem
(d) The hysteresis in a system occurs because of a change in temperature
(e) Hysteresis never occurs if the value to be measured is static

MTF Question 28

Regarding the cell salvage process:

(a) Blood can be salvaged from both suction and swabs
(b) A single-lumen large-bore (34 mm) suction tube is required

(c) High vacuum suction pressures (> 150 mmHg) are required
(d) Up to one-third of the red cell mass is lost during processing
(e) A consistent quality of packed red blood cells is produced

MTF Question 29

Which of the following statements regarding pharmacokinetic analysis are true?

(a) The rate constant may be expressed with units of seconds^{-1}
(b) The equation $\ln C = \ln C_0 - kt$ produces a straight line when plotted
(c) The time constant is equal to the inverse of the rate constant
(d) After one time constant, the value of the dependent variable will have fallen to approximately 37% of its initial value
(e) The rate constant represents the proportional change of the dependent variable per unit time

MTF Question 30

Cerebrospinal fluid (CSF) provides support and protection to the central nervous system. Which of the following statements concerning CSF are true?

(a) The total volume of CSF in an adult is approximately 150 mL
(b) The pH of CSF is comparable to that of plasma
(c) The formation rate of CSF is about 1.5 mL/minute
(d) Reabsorption of CSF by the choroid plexus is a passive process
(e) CSF has an increased glucose content compared to plasma

MTF Question 31

Which of the following statements regarding the distribution of drugs are correct?

(a) The vessel-rich body compartment comprises approximately 10% of total body mass but receives approximately 75% of the cardiac output
(b) The blood/tissue partition coefficient of a drug describes its relative distribution between body compartments at equilibrium
(c) Distribution and redistribution of drug between body compartments always uses blood as an intermediary
(d) Rate of uptake of drug into the body fat compartment is higher than into the vessel-rich compartment
(e) Drug distribution into body compartments always occurs down a concentration gradient

MTF Question 32

Regarding a vacuum-insulated evaporator (VIE), which of the following statements are true?

(a) A VIE should be sited in the open air more than 6 m from any combustible material
(b) A VIE should be large enough to provide 30 days of average oxygen consumption for the site it supplies
(c) A VIE is constructed of an inner carbon steel shell and an outer stainless steel shell separated by a vacuum
(d) The pressure in a VIE is greater at the bottom of the VIE than at the top of the VIE
(e) All oxygen leaving a VIE to enter the pipeline supply of a hospital is heated

MTF Question 33

Amiodarone is an acceptable first-line drug in the treatment of:

(a) Complete heart block
(b) Wolff–Parkinson–White syndrome
(c) Ventricular tachycardia
(d) Torsade de pointes
(e) Ventricular fibrillation

MTF Question 34

Regarding derived SI units, which of the following statements are correct?

(a) 50 degrees Celsius is equivalent to 323 kelvin
(b) Both joules and electron volts are measures of energy
(c) A coulomb (C) is the quantity of electricity transported in 1 second by 1 volt
(d) A pascal (Pa) is the pressure of 1 newton per square metre
(e) A force of 1 newton (N) will give a mass of 1 kilogram an acceleration of 1 metre per second

MTF Question 35

The analgesic ladder:

(a) Was originally championed by the World Health Organization to give guidance for cheap effective analgesia from acute pain in the developing world
(b) Recommends the use of adjuvant therapy only once strong opioids have failed to be effective
(c) Recommends that analgesics are given only as required to avoid adverse effects
(d) Recommends the use of a maximum of only three analgesic agents at any one time
(e) Has subsequently been shown to be 80–90% effective for cancer pain

MTF Question 36

Common side effects of amitriptyline at therapeutic doses include:

(a) Diarrhoea
(b) Agitation
(c) Hypertension
(d) Urinary retention
(e) Blurred vision

MTF Question 37

Regarding the circle system, which of the following are true?

(a) Increasing the length of the inspiratory and expiratory limbs will not alter the circuit dead space
(b) Circuit dead space will not be altered by failure of the expiratory unidirectional valve
(c) Placement of the fresh gas inlet between the patient and the expiratory unidirectional valve will allow re-breathing
(d) The adjustable pressure-limiting (APL) valve should be sited between the fresh gas inlet and the inspiratory unidirectional valve
(e) To maximise the lifespan of the CO_2 absorber, the CO_2 absorption canister should be located after the APL valve in the circle

MTF Question 38

Regarding standard external defibrillators, which of the following are true?

(a) Direct current is used to charge the defibrillator
(b) The key component within the circuit for storing of the electrical charge is the inductor
(c) The inductor ensures that the duration of the current flow is optimum
(d) The total current produced during a shock is about 35 A
(e) The shock delivered to the patient is AC energy

MTF Question 39

Which of the following statements about a sedative drug are true?

(a) Zopiclone is a benzodiazepine
(b) Plasma concentrations of zopiclone may be increased by concurrent administration of clarithromycin
(c) Zopiclone is suitable for long-term use as a night sedative
(d) Zopiclone is available as an intravenous formulation
(e) Zopiclone has active metabolites

MTF Question 40

Regarding atrial dysrhythmias:

(a) A wide QRS complex is an associated electrocardiographic feature of atrial fibrillation
(b) Atrial flutter waves are best visualised in the inferior leads
(c) Unlike atrial flutter, an isoelectric baseline is seen in atrial fibrillation
(d) The atrial rate in atrial fibrillation is typically in excess of 400 beats per minute
(e) With chronic atrial fibrillation, an enlarged left atrium would be expected on echocardiogram

MTF Question 41

Hyperkalaemia may be secondary to:

(a) Acute kidney injury
(b) Haemolysis
(c) Alkalosis
(d) β-Blockers
(e) High-dose glucocorticoids

MTF Question 42

Regarding capnography, which of the following are true?

(a) An upward slope in phase 3 may indicate uneven emptying of alveoli
(b) A difference of > 0.7 kPa between arterial carbon dioxide and end-tidal carbon dioxide is normal
(c) End-tidal carbon dioxide is always lower than alveolar carbon dioxide
(d) It is often inaccurate in neonates
(e) V/Q mismatch would decrease the difference between alveolar and end-tidal carbon dioxide

MTF Question 43

Regarding the measurement of pH, which of the following are true?

(a) pH is measured by the Severinghaus electrode
(b) pH is the logarithm to base 10 of hydrogen ion concentration measured in nmol/L
(c) Older samples will have a higher pH
(d) An arterial blood gas analyser will measure pH and base excess
(e) An increase in temperature will increase dissociation of acids

MTF Question 44

Calcitonin:

(a) Plays a major role in calcium homeostasis
(b) Is secreted by C cells
(c) Is secreted by the thyroid gland, lung and intestinal tract
(d) Is secreted by parafollicular cells
(e) Increases blood levels of calcium by activation of osteoclasts

MTF Question 45

Which of the following statements regarding mass are correct?

(a) Mass varies under conditions of differing gravity
(b) The SI unit for mass is the gram
(c) The unit for mass is based on a prototype held at Sèvres near Paris
(d) The term weight can be used interchangeably with the term mass
(e) Mass can be described as the gravitational force acting on an object

MTF Question 46

Glyceryl trinitrate:

(a) Is a pro-drug
(b) If administered as a patch, should be removed before defibrillation to avoid risk of explosion
(c) Principally exerts its antianginal effect by dilating the venous side of the circulation
(d) As an intravenous infusion may be limited in duration by the risk of developing methaemoglobinaemia
(e) Is contraindicated if the patient is found to have a failing left ventricle

MTF Question 47

Normal intracranial pressure (ICP) ranges from 5 to 15 mmHg. Regarding raised ICP, which of the following statements are correct?

(a) Headache associated with raised ICP is classically worse in the morning and relieved by stooping forward
(b) Cushing's reflex consists of marked hypertension and tachycardia
(c) Benign intracranial hypertension can lead to permanent blindness and is most common amongst young women
(d) Management of a patient with raised ICP includes encouragement of venous drainage by keeping patients slightly head-down
(e) Raised ICP may be a feature of Dandy–Walker syndrome

MTF Question 48

Regarding the Henderson–Hasselbalch equation:

(a) Provided the ratio of HCO_3^-/CO_2 remains constant, the pH of a system also remains constant
(b) The equation can be used to calculate the amount of acid or base required to make a solution a specific pH
(c) For a weak acid, if the pH is less than the pKa, molecules are more ionised
(d) The Henderson–Hasselbalch equation is based on the dissociation equation of carbonic acid
(e) The Henderson–Hasselbalch equation demonstrates why local anaesthetics are less ionised with increasing acidity

MTF Question 49

Regarding pipelines and medical suction, which of the following are true?

(a) All piped gases are supplied to theatre at 4 kPa
(b) The gas outlet at the wall consists of non-interchangeable screw-thread (NIST) connections specific for each gas
(c) The gas outlet at the wall consists of Schrader sockets specific for each gas
(d) Piped suction systems must have a minimum flow rate of 35 L/min
(e) Piped suction systems must generate a minimum of 7 kPa of negative pressure

MTF Question 50

Omeprazole:

(a) Activates the H^+/K^+-ATPase in parietal cells
(b) Is degraded by a low pH
(c) Leads to elevated gastrin levels
(d) As a sole agent for the treatment of duodenal ulcers heals the majority of patients within 4 weeks
(e) Is not used prior to caesarean section because of the risk of fetal bradycardia

MTF Question 51

Regarding acute kidney injury:

(a) A high urinary osmolality and sodium concentration would be expected in pre-renal injury
(b) The most common causes are pre-renal in origin
(c) Anuria is often observed in acute tubular necrosis
(d) In post-renal injury, a normal plasma creatinine suggests mild disease with minimal change in the glomerular filtration rate
(e) Pre-renal injury is associated with both conditions of volume depletion and overload

MTF Question 52

Which of the following statements about sevoflurane are true?

(a) Sevoflurane increases respiratory dead space
(b) Sevoflurane produces carbon monoxide when combined with dry sodalime
(c) Compound A production limits the use of sevoflurane in humans

(d) Sevoflurane is not suitable for use in head-injured patients since it raises the intracranial pressure

(e) Sevoflurane has a saturated vapour pressure of 20.9 kPa and a blood/gas partition coefficient of 0.69

MTF Question 53

Regarding safety features of the flowmeter bank on an anaesthetic machine, which of the following are true?

(a) Pressing the control valve spindle in will not alter gas flow rates
(b) Flowmeters can be interchanged to allow measurement of different gases
(c) The oxygen flow control knob must be octagonal in profile
(d) Oxygen flows into the back-bar manifold before (upstream of) any other gases
(e) The internal surface of the flowmeter tube is sometimes coated with gold

MTF Question 54

Which of the following statements correctly describe the principles of magnetism?

(a) A conductor of electricity can create a magnetic field without an external power source
(b) A magnet can create an electric current in a conductor without an external power source
(c) The unit of magnetic flux is the tesla
(d) The strength of the induced magnetic field in the galvanometer increases as the current through the wire increases
(e) The flow of blood generates an electric current when placed parallel to a magnetic field

MTF Question 55

Regarding conduction, which of the following statements are correct?

(a) Conduction is the most important route for heat loss during anaesthesia
(b) Gases are poor conductors of heat
(c) Heat loss via conduction is reduced by warming blankets
(d) Children and the elderly are at increased risk of hypothermia during anaesthesia
(e) Warming irrigating fluids reduces heat losses by conduction

MTF Question 56

Which of the following statements are correct regarding the measurement of functional residual capacity (FRC)?

(a) Helium is used for the gas dilution technique because of its low solubility in blood
(b) Body plethysmography depends on Boyle's law
(c) Measurements for the nitrogen washout technique begin at the end of maximal expiration
(d) The helium dilution method only measures communicating gas volume
(e) In a normal adult, body plethysmography overestimates FRC

MTF Question 57

The citric acid cycle:

(a) Is exclusive to carbohydrate metabolism
(b) Occurs in the cell cytoplasm

(c) Is initiated with citrate as its entry-point substrate
(d) Generates two adenosine triphosphate (ATP) molecules per molecule of glucose
(e) Is an aerobic process

MTF Question 58

Regarding the visual pathway:

(a) Axons from the nasal retina decussate in the optic tract
(b) Axons from the temporal retina decussate in the optic chiasm
(c) Axons from the temporal retina synapse in the contralateral lateral geniculate nucleus
(d) The primary visual cortex is located around the calcarine fissure
(e) The optic tracts relay information for eye movement to the superior colliculi

MTF Question 59

Regarding the resting membrane potential of cells:

(a) At rest, the cell membrane is more permeable to potassium than sodium
(b) The calculated Nernst potential for chloride is similar to the resting membrane potential
(c) The Nernst equation considers the effect of membrane permeability
(d) The resting membrane potential is less negative in acute potassium deficiency
(e) For nerve cells the resting membrane potential is –90 mV

MTF Question 60

Regarding the kidney, which of the following statements are correct?

(a) Renal blood flow can be estimated using para-aminohippuric acid
(b) Approximately 85% of inulin is cleared from the blood during one passage through the kidney
(c) Renal plasma flow can be estimated using para-aminohippuric acid
(d) The haematocrit must be known to calculate the effective renal plasma flow
(e) Inulin may be used to estimate renal plasma flow

SBA Question 61

A healthy 30-year-old runs the London Marathon. Immediately after completing the race serum lactate levels are measured and found to be 8.8 mmol/L. During exercise cellular respiration is both aerobic and anaerobic, leading to a build-up of lactate. Which ONE of the following processes in cellular respiration consumes oxygen?

(a) Metabolism of glucose to glucose-6-phosphate
(b) Metabolism of phosphoenol pyruvate to pyruvate
(c) Formation of acetyl-CoA from pyruvate and coenzyme A
(d) Formation of lactate from pyruvate
(e) Formation of water at the end of the electron transport chain

SBA Question 62

Which one of the following is NOT used to measure gas flow?

(a) Rotameter
(b) Pitot tube pneumotachograph
(c) Wright respirometer

(d) Wright peak flowmeter
(e) Fleisch pneumotachograph

SBA Question 63

During an in-theatre discussion with a consultant about the relevance of pKa, you are asked the following question. The pKa of lidocaine is 7.9, and at a pH of 7.4, 75% of the drug is ionised. The pKa of bupivacaine is 8.1. What percentage of bupivacaine is un-ionised at a pH of 7.4?

(a) 42%
(b) 37%
(c) 33%
(d) 26%
(e) 17%

SBA Question 64

The Association of Anaesthetists of Great Britain and Ireland (AAGBI) produced a checklist for anaesthetic equipment in 2004. As recommended by AAGBI, which of the following checks comes first?

(a) Check with a 'tug test' that each pipeline is correctly inserted into the appropriate gas supply terminal
(b) Check the breathing system to be employed
(c) Check all monitoring devices, particularly the oxygen analyser
(d) Check that alternative means to ventilate the patient is immediately available
(e) Check the operation of the flowmeters

SBA Question 65

In a patient on haemodialysis secondary to end-stage renal failure, which of the following drugs requires the least significant dose adjustment?

(a) Rifampicin
(b) Flucloxacillin
(c) Lithium
(d) Ranitidine
(e) Pancuronium

SBA Question 66

A significant reduction in physiological dead space occurs in a number of disease states. Which ONE of the following equations best describes measurement of physiological dead space? (V_D = volume of dead space, V_T = tidal volume, P_ACO_2 = alveolar partial pressure of CO_2, P_aCO_2 = arterial partial pressure of CO_2, P_ECO_2 = mixed expired partial pressure of CO_2)

Answers:

(a) $\dfrac{V_T}{V_D} = \dfrac{P_ACO_2 - P_ECO_2}{P_aCO_2}$

(b) $\dfrac{V_D}{V_T} = \dfrac{P_ECO_2 - P_ACO_2}{P_ECO_2}$

(c) $\dfrac{V_D}{V_T} = \dfrac{P_ACO_2 - P_ECO_2}{P_ACO_2}$

(d) $\dfrac{V_T}{V_D} = \dfrac{P_aCO_2 - P_ECO_2}{P_aCO_2}$

(e) $\dfrac{V_D}{V_T} = \dfrac{P_aCO_2 - P_ECO_2}{P_aCO_2}$

SBA Question 67

An 80-year-old gentleman is booked for an elective laparotomy. During your preoperative assessment you identify the need for careful temperature regulation during the procedure. Which of the following sites for temperature measurement would be the most accurate indirect measure of cerebral temperature for this patient?

(a) The rectum
(b) The nasal passage
(c) Peripheral skin
(d) The lower oesophagus
(e) The nasopharynx

SBA Question 68

Breathing system filters (BSFs) act as a barrier, protecting patients from particles and pathogens entering the respiratory system. Which one of the following is NOT a recognised mechanism used in BSFs?

(a) Interception
(b) Inertial impaction
(c) Electrostatic repulsion
(d) Diffusion
(e) Gravitational settling

SBA Question 69

Regarding the defibrillator, which ONE of the following statements is most correct?

(a) Stored energy can be calculated by ½ charge (millicoulombs) multiplied by the potential (volts)
(b) The coulomb is the capacitance of an object for which the electrical potential increases by one volt when one coulomb of charge is added to it
(c) Stored energy can be calculated by ½ charge (millicoulombs) divided by the potential (volts)
(d) The farad is the quantity of electric charge that passes some point when a current of one ampere flows for a period of one second
(e) The capacitor functions to smooth out the energy delivered to the patient

SBA Question 70

A 73-year-old, 61 kg female patient is admitted, intubated, to ICU following an aspiration of gastric contents post induction of anaesthesia. She is hypoxic with a PaO_2 of 6.1 kPa on FiO_2 of 1.0. She has had fluid boluses, metaraminol boluses, and now a noradrenaline infusion to manage worsening hypotension. You insert your cardiac output monitoring device and note the following data: heart rate 96 beats/min, blood pressure 68/46 mmHg, cardiac output 2.5 L/min, pulmonary capillary wedge pressure 20 mmHg, systemic vascular resistance 1400 dyn·s/cm^5. The ONE agent to best normalise this patient's haemodynamic variables would be:

(a) Noradrenaline
(b) Adrenaline
(c) Dobutamine
(d) Vasopressin
(e) Levosimendan

SBA Question 71

A 25-year-old woman who is 16 weeks pregnant is admitted to hospital with sudden onset of breathlessness and collapse. A transthoracic echocardiogram suggests a massive pulmonary embolus. An ECG is studied and shows sinus tachycardia with right axis deviation. The cardiac axis is likely to lie at which of these angles?

(a) −60 degrees
(b) +60 degrees
(c) +90 degrees
(d) +120 degrees
(e) −90 degrees

SBA Question 72

You are working as a ship's doctor in the tropics. The ship rescues a 40-year-old, 72 kg man from an island who was shipwrecked 2 days previously. He has had nothing to eat or drink for 2 days and the average daytime temperature has been 34 °C. He looks severely dehydrated but is conscious and cooperative. Which ONE of the following would be your fluid resuscitation of choice over the next 24 hours?

(a) Let him drink water freely
(b) Cautiously allow to drink water and administer 2000 mL of 5% dextrose solution intravenously over the next 24 hours
(c) Cautiously allow to drink water and administer 3000 mL of Hartmann's solution intravenously over the next 24 hours
(d) Prohibit oral fluids and administer 4000 mL of 0.9% saline solution intravenously over the next 24 hours
(e) Prohibit oral fluids and administer 5000 mL of dextrose saline solution intravenously over the next 24 hours

SBA Question 73

You are required to take over an emergency laparotomy in a 54-year-old, 80 kg male patient with a history of well-controlled hypertension who is otherwise previously fit and well. You insert an oesophageal Doppler probe and note the following haemodynamic observations: heart rate 103 beats/min, blood pressure 74/49 mmHg, cardiac output 4.1 L/min, flow time corrected (FTc) 290 milliseconds. Your initial management should be ONE of the following:

(a) Give a 200 mL intravenous colloid bolus over 5 minutes
(b) Give a 200 mL intravenous colloid bolus over 5 minutes and start an intravenous infusion of dobutamine
(c) Give a 200 mL intravenous colloid bolus over 5 minutes and start an intravenous infusion of metaraminol
(d) Give a 200 mL intravenous colloid bolus over 5 minutes and start an intravenous infusion of noradrenaline
(e) Start an intravenous infusion of gliceryl trinitrate

SBA Question: 74

During transfer of a ventilated patient to a regional neurosurgical unit there are several periods of cardiovascular instability requiring titration of the infusion of vasoactive medication. Which of the following statements is NOT a plausible explanation for the cardiovascular instability encountered during intermittent positive-pressure ventilation (IPPV)?

(a) Inspiration produces a decrease in venous return
(b) Inspiration produces an increase in left ventricular filling
(c) Right atrial compression produces a decrease in venous return
(d) Expiration produces an increase in right ventricular filling
(e) The secretion of atrial natriuretic peptide is reduced

SBA Question 75

You devise a new cardiovascular monitor that requires light to be shone through blood at two different wavelengths at which absorption of light is unaffected by the relative proportions of oxyhaemoglobin and deoxyhaemoglobin. Which ONE of the following combinations of light wavelengths would be best?

(a) 545 nm and 850 nm
(b) 530 nm and 815 nm
(c) 585 nm and 855 nm
(d) 570 nm and 905 nm
(e) 590 nm and 805 nm

SBA Question 76

Which of the following conditions is most likely to cause respiratory failure secondary to hypoventilation?

(a) Acute respiratory distress syndrome
(b) Acute exacerbation of asthma with peak expiratory flow rate 60% of that predicted
(c) Aspiration pneumonitis
(d) Acute inflammatory demyelinating polyneuropathy
(e) Acute pulmonary embolus

SBA Question 77

A patient arrives at preoperative assessment on a '100' fentanyl patch. This is equivalent to which of the following doses of oral morphine per day?

(a) 24 mg
(b) 60 mg
(c) 120 mg
(d) 240 mg
(e) 360 mg

SBA Question 78

In a 67-year-old previously fit and well female patient at the end of a laparoscopically assisted anterior resection, it is noted that the patient is still apnoeic 15 minutes after the volatile anaesthetic has been turned off. The patient had a rapid sequence induction. Expired gas desflurane concentration is only 0.74%. To aid your decision-making as to the cause of the delay, which ONE of the following would be most useful?

(a) Assess response to naloxone to exclude opioid excess
(b) Take the patient for a computerised tomogram of the head to look for a stroke
(c) Apply a BIS monitor to assess depth of anaesthesia
(d) Administer a dose of glycopyrrolate to reverse any residual muscle paralysis
(e) Provide supportive care with full anaesthetic monitoring but with no additional intervention for a further 15 minutes

SBA Question 79

You are asked to anaesthetise a patient for emergency laparotomy. The patient has an ASA score of III with a known significant history of ischaemic disease. Which ONE of the following statements about rapid sequence induction of anaesthesia in shocked patients is best supported?

(a) Etomidate causes less cardiovascular depression than other IV induction agents and is preferred for induction of anaesthesia in trauma
(b) A low pulse oximeter reading during induction of anaesthesia reliably suggests inadequate oxygenation
(c) Hypotension during induction should be diagnosed by palpating the pulse if an arterial line is not available
(d) If the patient cannot be intubated after two attempts with optimal head/neck positioning, he/she should be ventilated until spontaneous ventilation returns and then woken from anaesthesia
(e) Opioid drugs should not be used, as they cause a prolonged period of apnoea in shocked patients

SBA Question 80

You carry out an axillary nerve block using a nerve stimulator. Which ONE of the following statements is most accurate in describing the nerve stimulation you are carrying out as part of the block?

(a) Positive stimulation at a current of 0.2 mA suggests that injection of local anaesthetic will produce a reliable nerve block
(b) Positive stimulation at a current of 0.5 mA suggests that injection of local anaesthetic will produce a reliable nerve block
(c) The nerve stimulator should operate at 1–2 Hz to avoid damage to the nerve
(d) The duration of each stimulus generated by the nerve stimulator should be 1–2 ms to allow easy visualisation of the contractions
(e) Nerve stimulators used for monitoring neuromuscular blockade and those used for nerve blockade are interchangeable

SBA Question 81

Select the ONE option from the following that best describes current Resuscitation Council Guidelines on the use of sodium bicarbonate infusion during cardiac arrest:

(a) Sodium bicarbonate is contraindicated during the management of cardiac arrest
(b) Sodium bicarbonate should be administered routinely in cardiac arrest if a venous blood gas indicates a pH < 7.25
(c) Sodium bicarbonate is indicated if cardiac arrest follows toxicity from tricyclic antidepressant
(d) Sodium bicarbonate should only be administered if a cardiac arrest is complicated by hypokalaemia
(e) Sodium bicarbonate should be considered during any cardiac arrest lasting more than 30 minutes

SBA Question 82

In a small double-blind study of pain following minor surgery, patients were randomly allocated to receive either an analgesic or a placebo 1 hour preoperatively. The patients were then asked to rate their pain on a scale of 1 to 4, 1 being no pain and 4 being severe pain. Which of the following is the most appropriate statistical test for analysing the results?

(a) Mann–Whitney U-test
(b) Unpaired Student's t-test
(c) Fisher's exact test
(d) Chi-squared test
(e) One-way analysis of variance

SBA Question 83

Some basic knowledge of diathermy is required by the anaesthetist to ensure it is used safely. Which ONE of the following statements is true regarding diathermy?

(a) Bipolar diathermy uses a smaller power
(b) Diathermy usually uses direct current
(c) The frequency of the current is usually in the range of 0.5–1.0 Hz
(d) An alternating sine wave pattern is used for coagulation and a pulsed damped sine wave for cutting
(e) Pacemakers must be switched off before diathermy is used

SBA Question 84

A 40-year-old woman is in the recovery unit following a total abdominal hysterectomy. Her Hb is 6.5 and a blood transfusion is started. The patient becomes distressed, convinced that something terrible is about to happen, her blood pressure rapidly drops and the urine in her catheter is noted to be red. Which immune response is most likely to be occurring?

(a) Type 1 hypersensitivity reaction
(b) Type 2 hypersensitivity reaction
(c) Type 3 hypersensitivity reaction
(d) Type 4 hypersensitivity reaction
(e) Hyperacute host-versus-graft reaction

SBA Question 85

While you are sitting with a colleague waiting for a patient to wake from a volatile agent anaesthetic, your colleague examines the end-tidal agent concentration and states that the decline in value is occuring in an exponential fashion. Which of the following would be consistent with this assertion?

(a) A natural exponential function is a special form of linear change
(b) The time constant is equal to the half-life multiplied by 0.693
(c) After one time constant, the quantity has decreased by 37%
(d) The half-life is longer than the time constant
(e) The 'e' value is approximately equal to 2.718

SBA Question 86

A 40-year-old man known to have diabetes mellitus is admitted into hospital with collapse, and the following results are rapidly obtained from a venous blood gas: HCO_3^- 10; K^+ 3.6; Na^+ 132; Cl^- 104; glucose 20; lactate 3.1. These results enable calculation of:

(a) Anion gap
(b) Base excess
(c) Strong ion difference
(d) Osmolality
(e) eGFR

SBA Question 87

A 48-year-old 75 kg patient with polyarteritis nodosum is listed for an open reduction and internal fixation of a humeral fracture. The operation will take 90 minutes. He has been on oral prednisolone at 40 mg per day for the last 2 months. Which ONE of the following options demonstrates best management?

(a) Ensure the patient receives his normal oral prednisolone dose on the morning of the operation
(b) Ensure the patient receives double his normal oral prednisolone dose on the morning of the operation
(c) Ensure the patient receives his normal oral prednisolone dose on the morning of the operation and perform a brachial plexus block rather than a general anaesthetic
(d) Ensure the patient receives his normal oral prednisolone dose on the morning of the operation and during anaesthetic induction give 50 mg intravenous hydrocortisone
(e) Ensure the patient receives his normal oral prednisolone dose on the morning of the operation, during anaesthetic induction give 50 mg intravenous hydrocortisone, and give a further 25 mg intravenously every 8 hours for the next 24 hours

SBA Question 88

There are many methods of killing contaminating organisms. Which ONE of the following statements regarding decontamination, disinfection and sterilisation is correct?

(a) Disinfection is the removal of infected material
(b) Decontamination is the killing of infective organisms, not including spores
(c) Autoclaving uses dry heat
(d) Ethylene oxide is used for chemical sterilisation
(e) Prions may be destroyed by γ-irradiation

SBA Question 89

During a busy night shift a pizza is ordered by theatre staff. An anaesthetist walks into the coffee room and smells the pizza. Which of the following is the most potent stimulant of gastric juice under these circumstances?

(a) Histamine
(b) Acetylcholine
(c) Gastrin
(d) Somatostatin
(e) Adrenaline

SBA Question 90

As the anaesthetist on a mountain rescue team, you are asked if there are any risks involved with using Entonox in cylinders as a form of analgesia for a rescue operation. What would be the most appropriate response?

(a) Entonox should not be used at high altitude
(b) At a temperature of –10 °C it would be safer to use a cylinder supply of Entonox than a pipeline supply
(c) There is a risk of giving inadequate analgesia
(d) Entonox is not a useful form of analgesia
(e) There is a risk of giving a hypoxic mixture

Answers

Paper 1

Answers

1)	e	31)	c,d,e	61)	c
2)	a,d	32)	a	62)	a
3)	a,c,e	33)	a,b,c,e	63)	d
4)	a,b,d,e	34)	a,b,d,e	64)	d
5)	c,d	35)	b,c	65)	c
6)	a,b	36)	d,e	66)	b
7)	a,e	37)	d,e	67)	c
8)	c,e	38)	a,c	68)	b
9)	b,e	39)	a,b,d	69)	e
10)	b	40)	a,c,e	70)	b
11)	a,b,c	41)	a,c,e	71)	b
12)	a,d,e	42)	d,e	72)	d
13)	a,b,e	43)	c,e	73)	b
14)	a,c,d	44)	c,e	74)	e
15)	c,d,e	45)	d,e	75)	b
16)	b,c,d	46)	a,b,e	76)	b
17)	a,c,e	47)	c,e	77)	c
18)	a	48)	d	78)	b
19)	all false	49)	b,c	79)	b
20)	b,c,d,e	50)	b,c,d,e	80)	e
21)	b,d,e	51)	a,b	81)	b
22)	b,c	52)	b,d,e	82)	a
23)	a,c	53)	b,c	83)	b
24)	b,c,d,e	54)	d	84)	b
25)	a,c,d	55)	e	85)	d
26)	a,b,c,e	56)	b,d	86)	d
27)	a,d,e	57)	b,d,e	87)	a
28)	b,d,e	58)	e	88)	a
29)	a,c,e	59)	b	89)	b
30)	a,b,d,e	60)	a,b,d,e	90)	e

Paper 2

Answers

1)	b,c	31)	a,b,c	61)	e
2)	c,d	32)	a,d,e	62)	c
3)	b,e	33)	b,c	63)	e
4)	b,c,e	34)	a,b,d	64)	c
5)	a	35)	e	65)	a
6)	a,d	36)	d,e	66)	c
7)	b,e	37)	a,c,e	67)	d
8)	b	38)	c,d	68)	c
9)	a,b,c,d	39)	b,e	69)	a
10)	b,c	40)	b,d,e	70)	c
11)	b,c,e	41)	a,b,d	71)	d
12)	a,b,c,e	42)	a,c,d	72)	c
13)	c,d,e	43)	e	73)	a
14)	b	44)	b,c,d	74)	e
15)	c,d	45)	c	75)	e
16)	b	46)	a,c,d	76)	d
17)	b,d	47)	c,e	77)	e
18)	a,b,d	48)	a,b,d	78)	e
19)	a,c,e	49)	c,d	79)	c
20)	a,b,e	50)	b,c,d	80)	b
21)	d,e	51)	b,d,e	81)	c
22)	a,c	52)	a,b,e	82)	a
23)	a,b,c,e	53)	c,e	83)	a
24)	a,b,c,d,e	54)	b,d	84)	b
25)	a,b,c,e	55)	b,d,e	85)	e
26)	a,b	56)	a,b,d	86)	a
27)	e	57)	d,e	87)	e
28)	a,d	58)	d,e	88)	d
29)	a,b,c,d,e	59)	a,b	89)	b
30)	a,b	60)	a,c	90)	e

Explanations

Paper 1

MTF Question 1: Concepts of logarithms

Which of the following statements regarding logarithms are true?

a) $pH = \log_{10}[H^+]$
b) A solution with a pH of 6 is twice as alkaline as a solution with a pH of 3
c) A solution with a pH of 3 has 1/100th the acidity of a solution with a pH of 5
d) An acid with an H^+ concentration of 0.0001 M has a pH of 3
e) A solution with a pH of 8 is 100 times more acidic than a solution with a pH of 10

Answer: e

Short explanation

$pH = -\log_{10}[H^+]$. A solution with a pH of 6 is 1000 times more alkaline than a solution with a pH of 3 and a solution with a pH of 3 has 100 times the acidity of a solution with a pH of 5. If $[H^+] = 0.0001$ M, the pH is 4.

Long explanation

The pH scale is a logarithmic scale of acidity commonly used in anaesthesia and critical care. It ranges from zero (highly acidic) to 14 (highly alkaline). pH is defined as the negative logarithm to the base 10 of hydrogen ion concentration, i.e. $pH = -\log_{10}[H^+]$.

That the scale is logarithmic is key to answering this question correctly. For each one point increase in the pH scale, the concentration of hydrogen ions, and therefore acidity, changes by a factor of 10. Therefore, a solution with a pH of 4 is 10 times as acidic as a solution with a pH of 5, and 100 times more acidic than a solution with a pH of 6. Similarly, a solution with a pH of 6 is 1000 times less acidic than a solution with a pH of 3 and a solution with a pH of 3 has 100 times the acidity of a solution with a pH of 5.

The scale is relative in terms of $[H^+]$, so although a pH of 8 implies an alkaline solution, the number of H^+ ions still differs 100-fold from a solution with a pH of 10. Given that $pH = -\log_{10}[H^+]$, the pH of a 0.0001 M solution can easily be calculated. If $[H^+] = 0.0001$ M $= 10^4 = -\log(10^4) = pH\ 4$. More simply put, the pH is the number of times you need to move the decimal point to get 1 in this example.

Yentis S, Hirsch N, Smith G. *A–Z: Anaesthesia and Intensive Care an Encyclopaedia of Principles and Practice*, 3rd edn. Oxford: Butterworth–Heinemann, 2005; p. 409.

MTF Question 2: Etomidate

Which of the following statements about etomidate are true?

Answers:
a) The standard induction dose of etomidate is 0.3 mg/kg
b) Etomidate owes its anaesthetic activity to its action as an NMDA receptor antagonist
c) Etomidate is not suitable for use in major trauma since it raises intracranial pressure
d) Etomidate reversibly blocks the activity of the adrenocortical hormone 11β-hydroxylase
e) Etomidate has intrinsic analgesic activity equivalent to 5–10 mg of intravenous morphine

Answer: a,d

Short explanation

Etomidate enhances the action of GABA at $GABA_A$ channels; ketamine is an NMDA antagonist. Etomidate lowers cerebral blood flow and intracranial pressure. It has no intrinsic analgesic activity.

Long explanation

Etomidate is an imidazole derivative and an ester, which is presented as 0.2% solution in water and ethylene glycol or at the same concentration in a lipid emulsion. It is chiral with two enantiomers, of which only the R(+) isomer is biologically active. It is highly lipid-soluble and 75% protein-bound, making it sensitive to factors which change protein binding. The effect of a bolus of etomidate is terminated by redistribution of drug to peripheral tissues, and it is rapidly metabolised in the liver and by plasma esterases to inactive products. It works by enhancing the binding of GABA to $GABA_A$ receptors, and it has no intrinsic analgesic activity.

The standard dose for induction of anaesthesia is 0.3 mg/kg, producing anaesthesia in one arm-brain time. It has very little effect on the cardiovascular system, causing a very slight reduction in SVR, blood pressure and heart rate while preserving cardiac output. Indeed, the cardiovascular stability is so good that it has been recommended for use in hypovolaemic patients or those with poor cardiac function. Epileptiform activity is frequently seen on EEG and there is more excitatory muscle movement than is seen with barbiturates. It reduces cerebral blood flow, cerebral metabolic rate and intracranial pressure. It reduces tidal volume and respiratory rate, but to a much lesser degree than barbiturates.

Etomidate causes minimal histamine release and hypersensitivity is rare, but it does cause pain on injection and it seems to have a higher incidence of postoperative nausea and vomiting than other induction agents. It can also trigger a porphyric crisis in susceptible individuals. Most importantly, it blocks the function of the adrenocortical enzymes 11β-hydroxylase and 17α-hydroxylase, reducing corticosteroid and mineralocorticoid synthesis. This effect lasts for 3–6 hours after a bolus dose, but this is of little clinical significance in otherwise fit patients. However, when given as an infusion it causes profound adrenocortical blockade and has been shown to increase mortality; it is no longer licensed for use by infusion.

Pandit J. Intravenous anaesthetic agents. *Anaesth Intens Care Med* 2007; **9**: 154–9.
Smith T, Pinnock C, Lin T. *Fundamentals of Anaesthesia*, 3rd edn. Cambridge: Cambridge University Press, 2009.

MTF Question 3: Cylinder testing

Which of the following are required methods for testing medical gas cylinders in the UK?

a) Hydrostatic testing
b) Impact testing
c) Internal visual inspection
d) Ultrasonic testing
e) Tensile strength testing

Answer: a,c,e

Short explanation

Medical gas cylinders are hydrostatically tested every 5 years and both internally and externally inspected every 2.5 years. Details of these tests are stamped on a plastic ring that is placed around the neck of the cylinder.

Long explanation

Medical gas cylinders are subjected to rigorous testing to ensure a high level of safety. Testing in the UK should conform to British standards EN 1968 and 1802. During manufacture a proportion of medical cylinders are tested for tensile strength by being cut into strips. Every 5 years a cylinder must undergo hydraulic testing, and every 2.5 years a cylinder must be both internally and externally visually inspected.

External inspection is designed to look for signs of bulging, dents, thread damage, corrosion, etc., and if there is any suspicion of damage then an inspector may request a hydraulic test. Internal inspection uses an endoscope and, in addition, dental mirrors may be used to examine the area around the cylinder neck.

Hydraulic testing involves filling the cylinder with water and then placing it in a water-filled high-pressure chamber. The water pressure inside the cylinder is then increased to pressures of approximately 200–250 bar, which causes displacement of the water surrounding the cylinder as it expands. This displacement is measured, thus allowing cylinder expansion to be calculated, with an expansion of less than 0.02% being deemed acceptable. The results and date of testing are stamped on a coloured plastic disc that is then placed around the neck of the cylinder.

Other tests, such as impact testing and ultrasonic testing, have been and are still used in certain situations but currently do not form part of the regulated testing process.

MTF Question 4: Sodium

Regarding sodium in the human body, which of the following statements are true?

a) Sodium is key to the cellular co-transport (symport) or counter-transport (antiport) of virtually every other ion
b) It has a marginally higher concentration in cerebrospinal fluid than in plasma
c) Its Nernst potential is about −60 mV
d) Membrane-bound Na^+/K^+-ATPase extrudes three sodium ions for every two potassium ions that are taken up
e) Adult kidneys filter 25 mol of sodium a day

Answers: a,b,d,e

Short explanation

Sodium concentrations and transport are fundamental to the transmembrane fluxes of virtually every other ion in the human body. Sodium's Nernst potential is +60 mV.

Long explanation

One of the processes fundamental to human existence is the membrane-bound Na+/K+-ATPase pump. It expends adenosine triphosphate to actively remove sodium ions and admit potassium ions (in a ratio of 3 : 2) to the cell, resulting in the high intracellular potassium concentration and low intracellular sodium concentration common to all cells. This results in the negative resting membrane potential of all cells, without which the action potential of excitable cells would have no basis. This in turn means there is an electrochemical gradient encouraging sodium back into the cell, and this is exploited by membrane-bound transporters, which use the potential energy intrinsic to the gradient to move ions either into (via symports) or out of (via antiports) the cell.

The concentration gradient of ions on either side of the cell membrane is described by the Nernst equation:

$$E = \frac{RT}{zF} \ln \frac{[\text{ion}]_{\text{out}}}{[\text{ion}]_{\text{in}}} \quad \text{or} \quad E = 58 \log_{10} \frac{[\text{ion}]_{\text{out}}}{[\text{ion}]_{\text{in}}} \text{ mV}$$

where E is the membrane potential attributable to that ion, R is the universal gas constant (8.314 J/K per mol), T is the absolute temperature in K, z is the ionic valency of the ion concerned, F is Faraday's constant (96 500 coulombs/mol) and *out* and *in* refer to the extracellular and intracellular concentration of the ion concerned. Given that a number of the terms are constants, the formula can be simplified to the latter form shown.

Applying this to sodium gives a membrane potential of +60 mV. This is not achieved, because the membrane is impermeable to sodium and the resting membrane potential of potassium dominates. During an action potential, open sodium channels transiently render the membrane sodium-permeable, such that the positive membrane potential for sodium (+60 mV) is approached and the cell is temporarily depolarised.

The plasma concentration of sodium is 140 mmol/L. As the glomerular filtration is 180 L/day, it can be seen that 25 200 mmol of sodium (140 × 180) is filtered by the kidneys every day. 99.5% of this is reabsorbed along the length of the tubule; the exact quantity may be influenced by a number of factors.

MTF Question 5: Heparin-induced thrombocytopenia

Heparin-induced thrombocytopenia (HIT):

a) Is likely to require platelet transfusion
b) Usually presents with haemorrhage
c) Is mediated via an IgG autoantibody combined with platelet factor 4
d) Is most common with bovine heparin
e) Usually takes 36 hours to develop following a patient's first exposure to heparin

Answer: c,d

Short explanation

HIT rarely requires a platelet transfusion or presents with haemorrhage. The commonest clinical presentation is with thrombosis. Transfusion may make this worse. Typically HIT will develop 5 days after first exposure to heparin, but it may occur more quickly if the patient has had previous heparin within the last 3 months.

Long explanation

HIT is a condition in which patients administered heparin start to destroy their platelets. HIT is caused by the body raising an antibody to heparin. Heparin occurs naturally in the body, and it is thought that the body recognises administered heparin as being foreign, synthesising IgG (usually). The IgG combines in the circulation with platelet factor 4 (PF4), which then binds to the low-affinity immunoglobulin γ Fc region receptor II-a (FcγIIa receptor) on the platelet surface. This activates the platelets, which clump together, reducing the platelet count and potentially initiating thrombus formation.

HIT is most commonly found after administering bovine heparin. HIT is more likely to be produced in patients on unfractionated heparin, than low-molecular-weight heparin and typically occurs 5–14 days after treatment commenced. HIT may, however, occur within 1 day of administration if the patient has received heparin within the last month.

Most patients with HIT do not drop their platelet count enough to cause haemorrhage and are asymptomatic. HIT may be accompanied by thrombosis (HITT), and the most common presenting sign or symptom of HIT is usually development or extension of thrombus. Diagnosis usually initially involves full blood count screening. If a patient is thought to potentially have HIT, the risk can be stratified in the '4 Ts' scoring system by scoring points for the presence of Thrombocytopaenia, correct Timing of onset, the presence of Thrombosis and the absence of alTernative explanations. Laboratory testing would initially involve an ELISA test for the heparin–PF4 complex but, as this lacks specificity, a positive test would be followed by a functional test in which a sample of the patient's platelets and serum is assessed for serotonin release, which is a mark of platelet activation.

Management usually involves stopping heparin and introducing an agent to replace the heparin and manage additional thrombosis. Unfortunately, warfarin is associated with a higher incidence of warfarin necrosis in patients with established HIT, but some of the newer agents such as danaparoid have proven useful. Platelet transfusion is generally inadvisable, as it has been found to worsen the risk of thrombosis, and haemorrhage is rarely a problem in these patients.

Bennett PN, Brown MJ. *Clinical Pharmacology*, 10th edn. Edinburgh: Churchill Livingstone, 2008; p. 521.

MTF Question 6: Pharmacokinetic models

Which of the following statements regarding mathematical concepts about relationships and graphs are true?

a) In a multi-compartment pharmacokinetic model, drug can only be eliminated from the central compartment
b) A bi-exponential decline is seen in two-compartment models
c) Mammillary models have peripheral compartments that are directly linked to each other
d) The rate of transfer from the central compartment to a peripheral compartment is constant
e) In a multi-compartment pharmacokinetic model, a 'vessel-rich' peripheral compartment is where anaesthetic drugs have their effect

Answer: a,b

Short explanation
All administration/elimination occurs through the central compartment, which links the peripheral compartments in mammillary models. An 'effect-site' compartment of zero volume also equilibrates with the central compartment. Transfer between compartments is an exponential process. Two-compartment models have two exponential processes occurring (transfer to the peripheral compartment and elimination).

Long explanation
Single-compartment pharmacokinetic models are simple mathematical constructions allowing basic pharmacokinetic processes to be demonstrated and understood.

However, they cannot accurately represent actual drug behaviour, and models involving two or more compartments have more relevance to clinical situations. In multi-compartment models a central compartment (where drug is added to or removed from the system) is linked to one or more peripheral compartments. Drug moves from the central to the peripheral compartment(s) and back, and the rate of transfer in each direction is an exponential process governed by the concentration gradient and a rate constant which is different for each transfer process. The so-called 'effect-site' compartment is also linked to and equilibrates with the central compartment; however, it has zero volume and is therefore not part of the model itself.

All the processes of drug transfer between compartments and of drug elimination from the central compartment occur simultaneously, and the central compartment concentration at a given time (C) can be written as a function of all the relevant exponential processes. In a two-compartment model this would be $C = A \cdot e^{-\alpha.t} + B \cdot e^{-\beta.t}$, for example, where A and B are constants and α and β are the rate constants for the transfer of drug to the peripheral compartment and for elimination respectively. A graph plotting the log of central compartment drug concentration against time will therefore show a bi-exponential decline, with an initial rapid fall in the central compartment concentration as drug is distributed to the peripheral compartment followed by a slower terminal elimination phase.

A third compartment allows more complex modelling of drug distribution: the peripheral compartments have the characteristics of 'vessel-rich' or 'vessel-poor' tissue, allowing rapid distribution of drug to the former but slower distribution into a much larger volume for the latter. It is important to remember that these compartments are not intended to represent actual tissue compartments, however. In most models that are relevant to anaesthesia all the compartments are linked through the central compartment (mammillary models), although so-called 'catenary' models, where the compartments are directly linked, also exist.

Peck T, Hill S, Williams M. *Pharmacology for Anaesthesia and Intensive Care*, 3rd edn. Cambridge: Cambridge University Press, 2008.

MTF Question 7: Principles of cardiac pacemakers

Regarding the code used to classify artificial cardiac pacemakers, which of the following are correct?

a) The first letter denotes the chamber paced
b) The second letter denotes the chamber paced
c) The first letter denotes the chamber in which electrical activity is sensed
d) The third letter represents rate modulation
e) The fourth letter represents rate modulation

Answer: a,e

Short explanation
The second letter denotes the chamber in which electrical activity is sensed. The third letter refers to the response to a sensed electrical signal.

Long explanation
Artificial cardiac pacemakers have a variety of functions other than simple pacing of the heart muscle. They can have single- or dual-chamber functions, with one or two leads, respectively. In addition, there is the rate-modulation function, which allows adaptation of the pacing rate relative to the level of activity being undertaken. This means that the heart can meet the metabolic demand of the body during increased activity. There is also the possibility of defibrillation function for patients at high risk of tachyarrhythmias.

The first letter denotes the chamber paced; it can be A (atrial pacing), V (ventricular pacing) or D (dual-chamber pacing).

The second letter denotes the chamber in which electrical activity is sensed, and this can also be A, V or D. The letter O is used when pacemaker activity is not dependent on sensing electrical activity.

The third letter refers to the response to a sensed electrical signal. It can be T (triggering of pacing function), I (inhibition of pacing function), D (dual response) or O (where sensing function is absent).

The fourth letter represents rate modulation, and it can be R (rate-responsive physiological pacing) or O (no rate modulation).

The fifth letter represents multisite pacing and can be A (atrial), V (ventricular) or D (dual, pacing + shock)

Saraon TS. Pacemakers and implantable defisrillators. *Medscape Reference* 2011. Available online at emedicine.medscape.com/article/780825 (accessed 15 March 2012).

MTF Question 8: Diathermy

Regarding diathermy, which of the following are true?

a) The current density at the patient plate or neutral electrode is relatively high in monopolar diathermy
b) Monopolar diathermy is safer than unipolar diathermy for patients with cardiac pacemakers
c) Alternating current at frequencies between 0.5 and 1 MHz is used
d) The high frequencies used penetrate the myocardium
e) The amount of heat generated by diathermy is proportional to the square of the current divided by the area

Answer: c,e

Short explanation
The current density is low at the neutral plate in unipolar or monopolar diathermy. Unipolar and monopolar diathermy describe the same mechanism. The high frequencies used in diathermy do not penetrate tissue and pass directly over the myocardium.

Long explanation
Electrosurgical equipment is used during surgery to coagulate blood vessels, and to cut and destroy tissues by the heating effect of an electric current passed through them. The use of diathermy is not without significant risk to both patients and staff. An understanding of the basic principles allows a safe approach to the use of diathermy in clinical practice.

Alternating current with a frequency between 0.5 and 1 MHz is used. The cutting function requires a sine wave pattern and the coagulation function requires a damped or pulsed sine wave pattern.

Unipolar (monopolar) diathermy consists of a small tip where the current density and heating effect is high. The current flows through the patient to a neutral or patient plate, which is earthed. The patient plate is large so the current density and heating effect is negligible.

Bipolar diathermy equipment consists of two tips on a pair of forceps. The current passes across the field between the two tips to bring about heating. No patient or neutral electrode is required. Bipolar diathermy is preferable to unipolar if the patient has a cardiac pacemaker or central nervous system stimulator (spinal cord or deep brain), as the current is kept at the forceps tip and not passed through the body. This reduces the likelihood of current passing down the pacemaker or stimulator wire and exciting or damaging electrically conductive tissues. Bipolar diathermy is used for delicate surgery such as ophthalmic surgery and neurosurgery.

Al-Shaikh B, Stacey S. *Essentials of Anaesthetic Equipment*, 3rd edn. Edinburgh: Churchill Livingstone, 2007; pp. 217–18.

MTF Question 9: Pharmacophysiology and ageing

Regarding changes to the body that occur with ageing and might affect pharmacology:

a) Decrease in opioid receptor numbers and increase in receptor affinity are the main causes of toxicity due to opioids in the elderly
b) Reduced muscle bulk results in a prolonged effect for remifentanil
c) Bioavailability of drugs absorbed by the gastrointestinal system decreases by 50% by the age of 80 years old
d) As you age, you develop a relative decrease in body fat
e) As you age your volume of distribution (V_D) for water-soluble drugs decreases

Answer: b,e

Short explanation

Opioid toxicity is usually due to decreased plasma protein binding or decreased drug metabolism. Gastrointestinal absorption is well preserved in the elderly. As you age, total body fat decreases but proportionately your body fat increases, because your total body water decreases to a greater extent.

Long explanation

Many changes occur to the body as you age. These changes have a range of effects on how you respond to medications. Gastrointestinal absorption is generally preserved in the elderly. Hepato-portal blood flow and liver size decrease, along with the activity of hepatic enzymes. Hepatic drug clearance therefore decreases with age.

As you age, lean body mass, body fat and total body water all fall. The volume of distribution of most drugs is therefore reduced. This is particularly marked for drugs that are water-soluble, as the muscle mass reduces more than the fat mass. Elderly patients may be particularly sensitive to remifentanil, as a large proportion of its metabolism is catalysed by muscle-based esterases. Plasma albumin level is reduced as you age, and for plasma protein-bound drugs such as phenytoin this will lead to an increased proportion of unbound, active drug.

Renal clearance decreases as both glomerular filtration and tubular secretion deteriorate with age. Glomerular filtration rate falls by approximately 1% per year beyond the age of 30. Receptors also undergo changes as you age. Opioid receptors do decrease in number and increase in affinity, but the main reasons for increased sensitivity to these agents is usually either an increase in opioid unbound to plasma proteins or accumulation due to reduced metabolism.

Calvey N, Williams N. *Pharmacology for Anaesthetists*, 5th edn. Oxford: Blackwell, 2008; p. 92–3.

MTF Question 10: Cellular metabolism

Regarding cellular metabolism, which of the following statements are correct?

a) Aerobic metabolism of glucose is 80% efficient
b) 1 mol of glucose yields 38 mol of adenosine triphosphate (ATP) under aerobic conditions

c) The hexose monophosphate shunt produces carbon dioxide, ribose-5-phosphate and ATP

d) Glycogen is stored in skeletal muscle and the liver in approximately equal proportions

e) Under aerobic and anaerobic conditions, glycolysis generates a net gain of two ATP and two NADH

Answer: b

Short explanation

Aerobic metabolism of glucose only produces 42% of the energy available from 1 mol of glucose. Glycolysis generates two adenosine triphosphate (ATP) and two nicotinamide adenine dinucleotide (NADH) under aerobic conditions. Under anaerobic conditions, NADH is not produced. The hexose monophosphate shunt does not produce ATP. Skeletal muscle contains three times as much glycogen as the liver.

Long explanation

Glucose is the universal fuel for all cells and is the transportable form of carbohydrate throughout the body. The main pathways in carbohydrate metabolism are (1) glycolysis, (2) gluconeogenesis, (3) glycogenolysis and glycogenesis, and (4) the hexose monophosphate shunt. Under aerobic conditions, 1 mol of glucose generates 38 mol of ATP. As each molecule of ATP produces 7.6 kcal of energy, a total of 288 kcal is produced per 1 mol of glucose. When 1 mol of glucose undergoes combustion in a calorimeter, 686 kcal of heat is liberated. Therefore, aerobic metabolism of glucose has an efficiency of 42%.

Glycolysis breaks down glucose to pyruvate. Under aerobic conditions, two ATP molecules are used but four ATP and two NADH are generated. The NADH can then be used to yield further ATP. However, under anaerobic conditions, only a net gain of two ATP is produced and lactate accumulates.

Glycogen, a branched polymer of glucose, is the main storage form of carbohydrate in the body. A total of 325 g of glycogen is stored within skeletal muscle (75%) and the liver (25%). Storage of glucose as glycogen is highly efficient, with only 3% of the total energy available from glucose being utilised in the process of glycogenolysis.

The hexose monophosphate shunt, also known as the pentose phosphate pathway, is an alternative metabolic pathways for glucose. The activated form of glucose, glucose-6-phosphate, enters the pathways where fragments are transferred between pentoses. Carbon dioxide, ribose-5-phosphate and NADPH are produced. The NADPH acts as a reducing agent in tissues including the liver and adipose tissue.

Smith T, Pinnock C, Lin T. *Fundamentals of Anaesthesia*, 3rd edn. Cambridge: Cambridge University Press, 2009; pp. 453–5.

MTF Question 11: Adrenocortical hormones

Regarding the adrenal glands, which of the following are true?

a) The adrenal glands are retroperitoneal structures
b) The adrenal cortex develops from mesoderm
c) ACTH activates receptors in the zona fasciculata and the zona reticularis
d) The inner adrenal cortex produces the glucocorticoids
e) The adrenal glands are located inferior to the kidneys

Answer: a,b,c

Short explanation

The outer adrenal cortex produces the mineralocorticoids and glucocorticoids. The adrenal glands are usually located at the upper pole of each kidney.

Long explanation

The adrenal glands are a pair of triangular-shaped organs usually situated at the upper pole of each kidney, which is at the level of the 12th thoracic vertebra. They are surrounded by a connective tissue capsule and partially buried in an island of adipose tissue. Along with the kidneys they are retroperitoneal structures, and together they weigh 7–10 g.

Histologically and functionally the adrenal glands are divided into two parts. The outer cortex produces mineralocorticoids and glucocorticoids and consists of three separate layers. The inner medulla produces the catecholamines. The adrenal cortex consists of the zona glomerulosa, zona fasciculata and zona reticularis.

The adrenal cortex is stimulated to produce hormones by the neuroendocrine system, which originates in the hypothalamus, pituitary and kidney. The adrenal medulla is an extension of the sympathetic nervous system and is stimulated by sympathetic fibres from the thoracic sympathetic chain.

Bowen R. *Functional anatomy of the adrenal gland*. Available online at www.vivo. colostate.edu/hbooks/pathphys/endocrine/adrenal/anatomy.html (accessed 15 March 2012).

MTF Question 12: Heat radiation

Regarding infrared radiation:

a) Radiation is the most important route for heat loss from the body during anaesthesia
b) Radiation cannot transfer heat between two objects unless they are in contact with each other
c) Reflective shiny metallised plastic foil blankets should be used in theatre to prevent heat loss from radiation
d) Vasodilation increases heat loss by radiation
e) Radiation accounts for up to 50% of normal heat loss from the body

Answer: a,d,e

Short explanation

Radiation can indeed transfer heat between two objects that are not in contact. Reflective shiny metallised plastic foil blankets do prevent heat loss from radiation but should not be used in theatre because of an increased risk of burns and electric shock.

Long explanation

Heat energy can be transferred by electromagnetic radiation in the form of infrared radiation. This enables heat to be transferred across a vacuum in the absence of physical continuity. Radiation is indeed the most important route for heat loss from the body, accounting for 40–50% of losses.

A hot object will emit radiation over a spectrum of wavelengths predominantly in the infrared region. A hot object emitting radiation will lose heat energy and therefore cool down. However, if the heat is absorbed by another object, the temperature of the cooler object will rise. The rate of transfer between two objects is dependent on the temperature gradient between them and their surface characteristics: transfer of heat occurs from bright shiny objects to dark matt ones.

Reflective garments used in theatre do prevent heat loss by radiation but should be restricted to the use of caps, as heat loss from the head can be considerable. Heat loss in theatre can be reduced by covering the patient during transfer to and from theatre, by the maintenance of an ambient temperature between 22 and 24 °C and a humidity of about 50%, covering the patient with drapes, reflective garments and head coverings, and by warming all skin preparations and intravenous fluids. The use of warming blankets and warming of the bed will help to reduce losses.

Humidification of inspired gases reduces heat loss from the respiratory tract. Respiratory heat losses only account for about 10% of losses, but 8% of this loss occurs because of increasing the humidity of inspired air from 50% to 100%, and only 2% is because of warming. Therefore the use of dry inspired anaesthetic gases may contribute to hypothermia.

Davis PD, Kenny GNC. *Basic Physics and Measurement in Anaesthesia*, 5th edn. Oxford: Butterworth–Heinemann, 2003; pp. 103–4.

Smith T, Pinnock C, Lin T. *Fundamentals of Anaesthesia*, 3rd edn. Cambridge: Cambridge University Press, 2009; p. 740.

Yentis S, Hirsch N, Smith G. *Anaesthesia and Intensive Care A–Z: an Encyclopaedia of Principles and Practice*, 3rd edn. Edinburgh: Butterworth–Heinemann, 2008; p. 242.

MTF Question 13: Dexamethasone as an antiemetic

As an antiemetic, dexamethasone:

a) Is an effective rescue agent for postoperative vomiting
b) Should be administered at the beginning of the surgery
c) Is contraindicated for use in children
d) Should be used intraoperatively as an antiemetic with caution because of an increased risk of immunosuppression and wound infection
e) If given to an awake patient may produce uncomfortable perineal sensations

Answer: a,b,e

Short explanation
Dexamethasone is an extremely effective antiemetic for children. Dexamethasone does not produce any of the immunosuppression, when given as a single intravenous dose, that is found with longer courses of steroids.

Long explanation
The potent steroid dexamethasone is commonly used intravenously in a low dose as a first- or second-line agent during anaesthesia for the prevention of postoperative nausea and vomiting (PONV). Typically a one-off dose of 4 mg is given. This single dose has not been shown to produce significant adverse effects such as immunosuppression and poor wound healing.

In a 2006 Cochrane review of agents it was also found to have statistically significant rescue antiemetic properties, with a risk compared to placebo of 0.49 (95% confidence interval 0.41–0.58). Dexamethasone has been demonstrated in clinical trials to be an effective agent for the management of PONV in children.

Dexamethasone has been found to be most effective if given early on in the operation, unlike many other antiemetics such as the 5-HT$_3$ antagonists, which are best given 20 minutes before the end of the anaesthetic. A commonly reported adverse effect of dexamethasone when administered to awake patients is the sensation of uncomfortable perineal warmth.

Bolton CM. Prophylaxis of postoperative vomiting in children undergoing tonsillectomy: a systematic review and meta-analysis. *Br J Anaesth* 2006; **97**: 593–604.

Carlisle JB, Stevenson CA. Drugs for preventing postoperative nausea and vomiting. *Cochrane Database Syst Rev* 2006; (3): CD004125. Available online at mrw.interscience.wiley.com/cochrane/clsysrev/articles/CD004125/frame.html (accessed 15 March 2012).

MTF Question 14: Tocolysis

Regarding the use of drugs in pregnant women, which of the following agents are tocolytic?

a) Inhaled isoflurane
b) Intrathecal opioids
c) Intravenous glyceryl trinitrate
d) Intravenous magnesium sulphate
e) Epidural bupivacaine

Answer: a,c,d

Short explanation
Intrathecal opioids may cause uterine contraction, particularly in the presence of oxytocin, and epidural bupivacaine has not been shown to alter intrauterine pressure.

Long explanation
As well as understanding about the tocolytic agents that are deliberately given to pregnant women to delay delivery following premature onset of contractions, it is important for anaesthetists to understand about the tocolytic effects of the drugs they are likely to administer within obstetric anaesthesia. This is because effective uterine contraction is the most important physiological change that occurs following delivery to produce haemostasis, and interfering with this process may produce or worsen postpartum haemorrhage.

Volatile anaesthetic agents are tocolytic. Clinically significant uterine relaxation usually requires a dose above 1 minimum alveolar concentration (MAC). At a dose of 0.5 MAC volatile agents are not thought to significantly augment postpartum haemorrhage.

Both magnesium sulphate and glyceryl trinitrate are administered to pregnant women with pregnancy-induced hypertension, pre-eclampsia or eclampsia. Both of these agents are potent tocolytics and have been used as tocolytic agents. Glyceryl trinitrate works as a nitric oxide donor, and magnesium competes with calcium for uptake into the uterine muscle and increases intracellular cyclic AMP.

Experiments measuring intrauterine pressure in patients receiving epidural local anaesthetic do not demonstrate a change in uterine tone or coordination. Spinal opioids may actually promote uterine contraction, particularly in the presence of oxytocin. Fetal bradycardia may be seen after their administration.

MTF Question 15: Basic principles of ultrasound – Doppler effect

Which of the following are correct in relation to the Doppler effect?

a) The Doppler effect describes the phenomenon by which the amplitude of sound waves is altered if the source is moving in relation to the detector
b) The amplitude of sound waves is increased if the source of the sound is moving towards the detector
c) The frequency of sound waves is reduced if the source of the sound is moving away from the detector
d) The Doppler effect is used to measure blood flow velocity in arteries
e) The Doppler effect is used in obstetric practice when a fetal heart rate monitor is used

Answer: c,d,e

Short explanation
The Doppler effect describes the change in frequency of sound waves if the source of sound is moving in relation to the detector. The frequency is increased if the source is moving towards the detector and reduced if it is moving away.

Long explanation

The Doppler effect is used for many purposes in clinical medicine. Commonly, the Doppler effect allows the confirmation of flow within peripheral arteries using hand-held machines. The flow is represented by sound produced by the machine, and so the clinician can identify the presence or absence of flow. The Doppler effect is also used in conjunction with ultrasound imaging, where body structures are identified and flow is assessed. One of the commonest examples is during echocardiography, where flow across the heart valves and through the chambers of the heart is assessed. Flow can be assessed in most peripheral vessels as well as in the brain, where the circle of Willis can be scanned.

The Doppler effect is best explained by considering a series of waves travelling out from the centre of a circle in a pond. The frequency of the waves is related to the medium in which they are travelling and the speed at which they are travelling. As the waves moves further from the centre the distance between them increases and so the frequency of the waves reaching the periphery is less than the frequency nearer the centre. If a detector was in the periphery it would detect the frequency of the waves as they reached it, which remains constant. However, if the detector then started moving towards the source, the frequency would increase as the detector would be 'catching' the waves nearer to the centre, i.e. the source of the waves.

The Doppler effect is this change in frequency produced by motion of the target. When ultrasound waves are reflected back to a detector from a moving object their frequency changes in a similar manner. This difference in frequency is called the Doppler shift. The fetal heart rate monitor uses the Doppler effect, which detects the movement of the fetal heart during the cardiac cycle.

For more information see www.mrcophth.com/commonultrasoundcases/principleso fultrasound.html and www.centrus.com.br/DiplomaFMF/SeriesFMF/doppler/ capitulos-html/chapter_01.htm (accessed 15 March 2012).

MTF Question 16: Secondary hyperalgesia

Regarding the mechanism of secondary hyperalgesia:

a) Dorsal horn cells show reduced excitability in response to persistent pain
b) Excitation thresholds for mechanical stimuli in the dorsal horn cells fall
c) An increased area of receptive afferent input can be demonstrated
d) Secondary hyperalgesia is primarily due to a neuroplastic response in the dorsal horn
e) The presence of magnesium ions enhances the activity of NMDA receptors

Answer: b,c,d

Short explanation

Secondary hyperalgesia is a neuroplastic response that occurs in the damaged tissue and surrounding area. The dorsal horns cells become more excitable in response to persistent pain. Magnesium ions keep the N-methyl-D-aspartate (NMDA) receptors in an inactive state and therefore reduce their activity.

Long explanation

Hyperalgesia is the experience of an exaggerated response to a stimulus that we would normally expect to be painful. This can be further classified into primary and secondary hyperalgesia. Secondary hyperalgesia describes the pain we experience in the area surrounding the injury despite this area not having been directly injured. This is a good example of the flexibility or neuroplasticity of the nervous system. Persistent pain stimulates the dorsal horn cells via the nociceptive afferents. This results in an increased excitability of the dorsal horn cells, a reduction in excitation thresholds (specifically for mechanical stimulation) and an increased area receiving nociceptive inputs. In other words, pain is felt more quickly, with fewer stimuli and over a larger area than the initial injury.

One of the key excitatory neurotransmitters in this process is glutamate. There are several receptors in the dorsal horn to which it can bind. In acute pain it binds to the AMPA receptor, and in chronic pain to the NMDA receptor. Magnesium ions reduce the NMDA receptor activity by blocking them in an inactive state. Activation of AMPA by glutamate in acute pain releases the magnesium block, increasing the NMDA receptor activity and excitability of the neurones.

Substance P, brain-derived neurotrophic factor (BDNF) and increased intracellular calcium via NMDA-linked calcium channels are all essential components of the neuroplastic phenomenon of secondary hyperalgesia.

Smith T, Pinnock C, Lin T. *Fundamentals of Anaesthesia*, 3rd edn. Cambridge: Cambridge University Press, 2009; pp. 412–32.

MTF Question 17: Laryngoscopes

Which of the following statements are true regarding laryngoscope blades?

a) The standard Macintosh laryngoscope blade is available in four sizes
b) The Magill laryngoscope blade is curved
c) The Macintosh laryngoscope blade should be placed anterior to the epiglottis in the vallecula during laryngoscopy for intubation
d) The Miller laryngoscope blade should be placed anterior to the epiglottis in the vallecula during laryngoscopy for intubation
e) A 'left-sided' version of the Macintosh laryngoscope blade is available

Answer: a,c,e

Short explanation
The Miller and Magill laryngoscope blades are straight blades, which should be placed posterior to the epiglottis during laryngoscopy for intubation. The Macintosh curved laryngoscope blade is the most commonly used in the UK and is available in a 'left-sided' version for patients with right-sided facial deformity.

Long explanation
Direct-view laryngoscopes were invented in the late 1800s. Before this, doctors and surgeons used mirrors and other tools to view the larynx. There are many different designs of blade, which are widely available to assist in direct laryngoscopy. Laryngoscopes are made up of the blade and a handle. The handle usually houses the power source (batteries) and is also available in different sizes. An electrical connection exists between the handle and the blade, which is clipped on to the handle. The bulb or fibreoptics is attached to the blade to provide the light source.

The most commonly used laryngoscope blade in the UK is the curved Macintosh blade. The curved blade is placed in the vallecula, where the epiglottis and other structures are lifted up and forward to expose the vocal cords. The Miller and Magill blades are versions of many straight blades available for use. Other versions include the Wisconsin and Soper blades.

The straight blades are often preferred in children, as the epiglottis is larger and floppier. The straight blade is placed posterior to the epiglottis, where it is lifted out of the way of the vocal cords. Special paediatric versions exist, such as the Robertshaw, Seward and Oxford infant laryngoscope blades.

For pictures see www.laryngoscopeblades.com/laryngo-conv.htm and www.adair.at/
eng/museum/equipment/laryngoscopes (accessed 15 March 2012).
Al-Shaikh B, Stacey S. *Essentials of Anaesthetic Equipment*, 3rd edn. Edinburgh: Churchill
Livingstone, 2007; pp. 98–9.

MTF Question 18: Narcotic analgesia in children

Regarding narcotic analgesia in children:

a) An 8-year-old child may be prescribed a patient-controlled analgesia (PCA) device
b) Parent-controlled analgesia (PrCA) is rarely used because it is likely to produce apnoea or excessive narcosis
c) Neonates do not require opioids
d) All children under 10 years old receiving an opioid infusion should have continuously monitored pulse oximetry
e) Nasal fentanyl is not recommended in children under the age of 10 because of the risk of apnoea

Answer: a

Short explanation
PrCA has been shown to have a good safety profile and if well managed is not likely to produce apnoea. Neonates may require opioids. There are no national guidelines on pulse oximetry use and some centres would consider observations alone acceptable in low-risk patients. Intranasal fentanyl has been safely used in infants.

Long explanation
If simple analgesics and local anaesthetic administered intraoperatively provide insufficient analgesia for a child, it may be necessary to use narcotic analgesics. This goes right across the age range for paediatric care. It used to be thought that neonates had an immature perception of pain and high circulating endogenous endorphins and therefore did not require opioids. Data on increased risk of side effects from under-analgesia such as intercerebral bleeding have now changed this attitude. Neonates may sometimes require opioids.

Patient-controlled analgesia (PCA) has been extensively studied in paediatric care. Efficacy is better than intermittent nurse-administered opioid boluses. Children as young as 6 years old may benefit from PCA. A good cut-off test is if the child can comprehend that if they push the button the pain will be less. This acts as an effective screen to determine whether the child is mature enough to use a PCA.

Some studies have reported the use of parent-controlled analgesia (PrCA), with very high parental satisfaction scores and no reports of excessive narcosis or apnoea. To achieve this, PrCA does require diligent monitoring and appropriate education of the parent about the technique. Therefore, under correctly managed circumstances it is not likely to produce apnoea or excessive narcosis. The concern with PrCA is that it removes the in-built safety feature within PCA. With a PCA, the adequately or mildly over-narcotised patient will no longer press the button. The anxiety with PrCA is that an anxious parent, concerned that the child is in pain, overdoses the child, leading to hypoventilation. This has been reported in the literature with some fatal outcomes. These cases were generally in opioid-naive patients with inadequately informed or supported parents and poor or absent monitoring.

With all opioid infusions, the main risk of death is hypoventilation. It would make sense to monitor all patients receiving such infusions. The problems with pulse oximetry include discomfort, repeated detachment and annoying false-positive alarms. There is no national guideline that all paediatric patients should have pulse oximetry monitored if receiving opioids, and local policy needs to be followed. Many units have a pragmatic approach, monitoring initial therapy, recording regular observations such as respiratory rate to detect a trend towards overdosing and a screening system for picking up at-risk patients who will need continuous oximetry from the outset.

Intranasal fentanyl is a new delivery system that has now been widely trialled in children. Emergency departments have squirted syringes of diamorphine up children's noses for some time. However, due to supply problems with diamorphine, intranasal fentanyl has been introduced to fill the gap. There are numerous studies in the literature, with many including children down to 6 months age or 10 kg body weight. The safety profile and efficacy for this system are generally excellent, and it would certainly be safe enough for use in children less than 10 years old.

Choi SH, Lee WK, Lee SJ, *et al.* Parent-controlled analgesia in children undergoing cleft palate repair. *J Korean Med Sci* 2008; **23**: 122–5. Available online at jkms.org/DOIx.php?id=10.3346/jkms.2008.23.1.122 (accessed 15 March 2012).

Monitto CL, Greenberg RS, Kost-Byerly S, *et al.* The Safety and efficacy of parent-/nurse-controlled analgesia in patients less than six yeas of age. *Anesth Analg* 2000; **91**: 573–9. Available online at www.anesthesia-analgesia.org/content/91/3/573.full (accessed 15 March 2012).

MTF Question 19: Cardiac output measurement

Which of the following statements regarding the measurement of cardiac output using thermodilution are correct?

a) The cold solution should be injected into the right ventricle
b) Injection is performed during the inspiratory phase of the breathing cycle
c) The graphical data obtained has temperature increasing on the y axis
d) Semi-logarithmic data is required for the calculation of cardiac output
e) The cardiac output is the area under the temperature–time graph

Answer: all false

Short explanation
The cold solution is injected into the pulmonary artery during the expiratory phase of breathing. The plotted data is linear, not semi-logarithmic, with temperature decreasing along the y axis. Calculation of the cardiac output requires mathematical formulae; it cannot simply be obtained from the area under the graph.

Long explanation
Cardiac output measurement by thermodilution has evolved as a common technique for use in the operating theatre or intensive care unit. Although the use of thermodilution via a pulmonary artery catheter is the gold-standard technique for determining cardiac output in critically ill patients, its use is becoming less commonplace owing to the adverse events associated with the technique and the lack of data supporting improved outcomes with its use.

When performing the thermodilution technique, a cold solution of approximately 10 mL is injected into the appropriate port of the pulmonary artery catheter. The fluid enters the pulmonary artery and the flow of blood carries it to a thermistor placed more distally along the catheter, but still within the pulmonary artery, where the temperature is recorded. The injection should be performed at the end of expiration to avoid the haemodynamic changes associated with inspiration, particularly notable if patients are subjected to positive-pressure ventilation. A plot of temperature against time is then made (which need not be semi-logarithmic when using thermodilution) on computer. The temperature is plotted on the y axis, with a lower temperature being found furthest from the bisection with the x axis. Cardiac output is then calculated from the area under the graph by the application of the Stewart–Hamilton equation. It is not simply the area under the graph.

Harvey S, Harrison DA, Singer M, *et al.* Assessment of the clinical effectiveness of pulmonary artery catheters in management of patients in intensive care (PAC-Man): a randomised controlled trial. *Lancet* 2005; **366**: 472–7.

Yentis S, Hirsch N, Smith G. Cardiac output measurement. In: *A–Z of Anaesthesia and Intensive Care: an Encyclopaedia of Principles and Practice*. Edinburgh: Butterworth–Heinemann, 2005; p. 93.

MTF Question 20: Insulin

Regarding insulin:

a) Some intermediate-acting insulins should not be used in patients with known allergy to heparin
b) The majority of insulin used in the UK is structurally human insulin
c) Complexing insulin with zinc decreases the rate at which it is absorbed
d) 50% of subcutaneously injected insulin enters the circulation by local absorption across the capillary wall and 50% via the lymphatics
e) Some insulin preparations become shorter-acting during an acidosis

Answer: b,c,d,e

Short explanation
Patients with protamine allergy should avoid some insulins such as isophane as the insulin is complexed with protamine.

Long explanation
Of the 2.3 million people with diabetes mellitus in the UK, around 10% have type 1 diabetes and require insulin therapy. Even though insulin may be administered intravenously in diabetic emergencies or by inhalation if injections are not an option, the vast majority of insulin is administered as a subcutaneous injection.

Insulin is made up of 51 amino acids and has a molecular weight of 5808 Da. Molecules with a size >16 000 Da are primarily absorbed by the lymphatics. Experiments on lymphatic cannulated sheep would indicate that around 50% of insulin deposited in the interstitial space is transported to the systemic circulation via the lymphatics. Following its initial use in 1922, insulin was prepared and purified from animal sources. The first genetically engineered human insulin was synthesised in 1977, and now the majority of insulin used in the UK is structurally human.

Various tactics have been used to make a dose last longer. Some insulins are complexed with zinc (e.g. insulin zinc suspension) or protamine (e.g. isophane) to decrease absorption rate. Protamine allergy (rather than heparin allergy) would therefore be an issue. Some are turned into crystalline form to slow absorption. A drug such as insulin glargine takes advantage of the drug's pKa to ensure the drug is soluble in the acid conditions in which it is stored, but precipitates in the relatively more alkaline tissues at physiological pH. Such a drug would be shorter-acting in the presence of an acidosis, but the true relevance of this is debatable.

Charman SA, McLennan DN, Edwards GA, Porter CJ. Lymphatic absorption is a significant contributor to the subcutaneous bioavailability of insulin in sheep. *Pharm Res* 2001; **18**: 1620–6. Available online at www.springerlink.com/content/nn812t2h6k9319h4/fulltext.pdf (accessed 15 March 2012).

Neal MJ. *Medical Pharmacology at a Glance*, 6th edn. Oxford: Wiley-Blackwell, 2009; p. 79.

MTF Question 21: Coaxial breathing systems

Regarding coaxial breathing systems, which of the following are true?

a) The use of a coaxial breathing system will allow the use of a lower fresh gas flow (FGF) without re-breathing compared to the non-coaxial equivalent system

b) The coaxial form of the Mapleson D breathing system is known as the Bain circuit
c) The diameter of the external breathing hose on a coaxial system is similar to the diameter of the breathing hose in a non-coaxial system
d) Disconnection of the inner lumen of a Bain circuit may cause a rise in the inspired CO_2 concentration
e) The Lack circuit is functionally similar to a Mapleson A system

Answer: b,d,e

Short explanation
A coaxial breathing system is functionally similar to its non-coaxial equivalent, and will not allow reduced FGF. The inner lumen of a coaxial system will cause increased resistance to ventilation, so the diameter of the external lumen is increased.

Long explanation
In a Mapleson A system, the adjustable pressure-limiting (APL) valve and scavenging is at the patient end of the system, which is inconvenient and applies traction to the patient's airway. With a Mapleson D system, the FGF flows into the patient end of the system, which again is inconvenient.

The coaxial equivalents were designed to reduce these inconveniences. Ideally, the APL and FGF would be at the machine end of the circuit to reduce the weight on the patient's airway and make it easier for the anaesthetist to control. An inner lumen was added to the breathing circuit. The coaxial Mapleson A system is known as a Lack circuit, and the inner lumen carries exhaled gas away from the patient towards the APL. A coaxial Mapleson D is known as a Bain circuit, and the inner lumen carries FGF so that it is inserted into the breathing system at the patient end.

The coaxial systems are functionally similar to their non-coaxial equivalents – they behave in the same manner during mechanical and spontaneous ventilation, and require similar FGFs. The addition of the inner tube introduces additional resistance to breathing by reducing the effective diameter. To overcome this, the diameter of the external lumen is increased. The integrity of the inner lumen of the Bain circuit is critical to its effective function. If the inner lumen is disconnected, the FGF will enter the breathing circuit at the machine end, just next to the APL. This means that the flushing effect of the FGF is lost, and the whole system becomes dead space. Significant re-breathing will occur and the inspired CO_2 will rise.

Davey A, Diba A. Breathing systems and their components. In: *Ward's Anaesthetic Equipment*, 5th edn. Philadelphia, PA: Saunders, 2005; pp. 131–63.

MTF Question 22: Furosemide

Furosemide:

a) Is not as effective a diuretic as a thiazide in patients with chronic kidney disease
b) Is more likely to cause deafness in patients with nephrotic syndrome
c) Reduces both cardiac preload and afterload before causing a diuresis
d) Potentiates the nephrotoxicity of gentamicin
e) Causes a diuresis that is enhanced by the co-administration of non-steroidal anti-inflammatory drugs

Answer: b,c

Short explanation

Furosemide is effective in patients with impaired renal function, whereas the thiazides are not. They potentiate the ototoxic effects of gentamicin and are less effective diuretics in combination with non-steroidal anti-inflammatory drugs.

Long explanation

Furosemide is a loop diuretic, interfering with the powerful concentrating capacity of the loop of Henle. The loop diuretics, in general, are effective in patients with impaired renal function, whereas the thiazides are not.

Ototoxicity may be caused, particulary by high doses given intravenously. An additional risk factor is the presence of hypoproteinaemia, which is a common complication of nephrotic syndrome. Furosemide potentiates the nephrotoxic effects of cephalosporins and the ototoxic effects of aminoglycosides.

Non-steroidal anti-inflammatory drugs inhibit renal prostaglandin, causing Na^+ to be retained, which reduces the diuresis caused by furosemide. Furosemide is an arteriolar and venous vasodilator and has been found to reduce both preload and afterload in a time frame that precedes the onset of a significant diuresis.

Bennett PN, Brown MJ. *Clinical Pharmacology*, 10th edn. Edinburgh: Churchill Livingstone Elsevier, 2008; pp. 481–6.

Neal MJ. *Medical Pharmacology at a Glance*, 6th edn. Oxford: Wiley-Blackwell, 2009; pp. 34–5.

Peck T, Hill S, Williams M. *Pharmacology for Anaesthesia and Intensive Care*, 3rd edn. Cambridge: Cambridge University Press, 2008; pp. 307–8.

MTF Question 23: Enzyme induction and inhibition

Which of the following statements regarding enzyme induction and inhibition are correct?

a) Phenytoin increases the metabolism of certain drugs, including tricyclic antidepressants
b) Induction of an enzyme is caused solely by increased gene expression
c) Metronidazole enhances the toxicity of ethanol
d) Aminophylline has an increased duration of action in smokers
e) Rifampicin enhances the toxicity of ethanol

Answer: a,c

Short explanation

Enzyme induction can be caused by increased gene expression, decreased enzyme breakdown, or allosteric modulation. Phenytoin, rifampicin and smoking induce liver enzymes and reduce the duration, effectiveness and toxicity of the other drugs mentioned. Metronidazole is an enzyme inhibitor and causes a build-up of acetaldehyde after drinking alcohol.

Long explanation

Enzyme activity can be increased (induction) or decreased (inhibition) by drugs. This may be due to an increase in the amount of enzyme (due to changes in gene expression or enzyme metabolism), or it may be due to allosteric modulation, a change in the three-dimensional structure of the enzyme caused by the binding of another molecule. Allosteric modulation can work either through altering the binding of the substrate to the enzyme or through changing the ability of the enzyme to perform its function.

Alterations in enzyme activity can have many effects, particularly if the enzyme is involved in drug metabolism. Many enzymes from the cytochrome P450 (CYP) superfamily metabolise more than one drug entity, and inhibition or induction of these enzymes by certain drugs can lead to wide variations in drug levels.

Phenytoin is an example of an enzyme inducer, and it will increase the metabolism (and hence decrease the effective levels) of digoxin, thyroxine and tricyclic antidepressants. Smoking and rifampicin are also classic examples of enzyme inducers, reducing the duration of action and toxicity of other agents, including aminophylline and alcohol, respectively. Metronidazole is an enzyme inhibitor and has a marked effect on aldehyde dehydrogenase, leading to the build-up of acetaldehyde after the consumption of alcohol.

Yentis S, Hirsch N, Smith G. *Anaesthesia and Intensive Care A-Z: an Encyclopaedia of Principles and Practice*, 4th edn. Edinburgh: Butterworth–Heinemann, 2009.

MTF Question 24: Density and viscosity of gases

Which of the following are true?

a) The SI unit of dynamic viscosity is a newton·second/metre
b) The viscosity of blood is dependent on flow rate
c) A thixotropic material is a material that becomes less viscous over time when it is agitated or otherwise stressed
d) The dynamic viscosity of a gas is independent of pressure
e) The relationship between viscosity and temperature and pressure only holds true for those fluids and gases that exhibit 'Newtonian' properties

Answer: b,c,d,e

Short explanation

The SI unit of dynamic (or absolute) viscosity is the pascal-second (Pa·s), equivalent to newton·second/metre^2. Blood is a non-Newtonian fluid so its viscosity is flow-dependent. Dynamic viscosity is pressure-independent, and the viscosity of blood increases with age.

Long explanation

Dynamic or absolute viscosity is a measure of the resistance of a fluid or gas to flow. It is measured using a viscometer or rheometer. Viscosity essentially describes the internal friction of a moving fluid or gas. The greater the viscosity, the greater the resistance to motion of the particular substance, owing to greater internal forces (e.g. van der Waal forces) between the individual molecules. These internal forces generally act between layers of the fluid (and to a certain extent, gas) moving at different velocities.

The SI unit of dynamic (or absolute) viscosity is the pascal-second (Pa·s), equivalent to N·s/m^2. Kinematic velocity is defined as the dynamic velocity of a substance divided by its density. A thixotropic substance is a substance that becomes less viscous over time when agitated or otherwise stressed. If the opposite occurs, this is known as a rheopectic material.

For a gas, viscosity decreases as its temperature increases but its viscosity is independent of pressure. The relationship between viscosity and temperature and pressure only holds true for those fluids and gases that exhibit 'Newtonian' properties, i.e. substances that will always flow irrespective of forces acting upon them (e.g. crystalloid solutions and water). Another important characteristic property of Newtonian substances is that their viscosity is independent of the rate at which the substance is flowing (be it a gas or liquid).

Blood is an example of a non-Newtonian fluid (so its viscosity varies with flow rate) and its viscosity depends largely on haematocrit. Blood viscosity is higher in cigarette smokers (caused, in part, by the increase in haematocrit). Blood viscosity is also increased by volatile anaesthetic agents, but not propofol.

MTF Question 25: Other units relevant to anaesthesia

Which of the following statements are correct with regard to units of measurement?

a) A tall adult male with a weight of 686 N would not be considered obese
b) One kilocalorie is equal to 4.2 joules
c) Pipeline pressure on the anaesthetic machine is equal to 3000 mmHg
d) Normal body temperature is approximately equal to 97.8 °F
e) A mean arterial blood pressure of 109 cmH$_2$O is not compatible with life

Answer: a,c,d

Short explanation
The kilocalorie, often confusingly referred to as the calorie, is a unit of energy that is most commonly used to quantify the amount of energy in food. One kilocalorie is equal to 4.2 kJ, not 4.2 J. A mean arterial blood pressure of 109 cmH$_2$O is equal to 80 mmHg and is therefore compatible with life!

Long explanation
There are a number of non-SI units that are still in common use in medicine, although there is a move to stop using them entirely.

The recognised SI unit for pressure is the pascal (Pa) and the unit for temperature is the kelvin (K). There are a number of units of pressure, some of which are used for convenience. The pressure unit of bar is commonly used to quote high pressure values such as pipeline gas pressure at the anaesthetic machine, which is usually 4 bar, which is equal to 3000 mmHg. One atmosphere of pressure (1 atm) is equal to 101.325 kPa, and this should not be confused with a bar of pressure, which is equal to 100 kPa or 750 mmHg. Millimetres of mercury (mmHg) is still in common use when quoting arterial blood pressure.

It is technically incorrect to quote weight in kilograms. Mass is quoted in kilograms, and the weight is the gravitational force on an object. Acceleration due to gravity on the Earth is equal to 9.81 m/s^2 (often quoted as 10 for convenience). An adult male with a weight of 686 N has a mass of 70 kg.

Other units for expressing temperature include degree Celsius (°C), degrees Fahrenheit (°F), degrees Reaumur and Rankine. Of these, the degree Celsius (°C) and degree Fahrenheit (°F) are in common use, although Fahrenheit is more commonly used in the USA. To convert Fahrenheit to Celsius, subtract 32, divide the answer by 9 and then multiply by 5. This calculation can be reversed to convert Celsius to Fahrenheit. Normal body temperature is approximately equal to 36.6 °C, 97.8 °F, or 309.8 K.

A page on metric conversions is available online at www.metric-conversions.org (accessed 15 March 2012).

MTF Question 26: Labelling of valve blocks

Regarding a valve block that is attached to a medical gas cylinder:

a) There is a metal seal between the valve and cylinder that will melt at 70 °C, thus reducing the risk of explosion
b) It is marked with the tare weight of the cylinder
c) It is marked with the chemical symbol of the gas contained in the cylinder
d) It is marked with the name of the gas contained in the cylinder
e) There is a unique serial number stamped on each valve block

Answer: a,b,c,e

Short explanation

A valve block is marked with the chemical symbol of the cylinder gas, a unique serial number and the tare weight. The name of the gas is on the valve block label (not the valve block).

Long explanation

The valve block screws into the open end of a cylinder. It is marked with a unique serial number and the tare weight of the cylinder to which it is attached. In the UK there is a metal seal placed between the valve block and cylinder neck made of Wood's metal (otherwise known as Lipowitz's alloy). This is a eutectic alloy made up of bismuth, lead, tin and cadmium that will melt at 70 °C, thus allowing cylinder contents to escape if external temperatures rise; this reduces the risk of potential explosion.

The valve block is also marked with the symbol of the gas the cylinder contains. A label is also attached to the body of the cylinder. This contains the content name and chemical symbol, content licence number, hazard warning signs, the volume of the cylinder in litres, storage and handling instructions, and the maximum safe cylinder pressure. A coloured plastic disc containing information regarding the test is added around the neck of the cylinder each time a cylinder is tested.

MTF Question 27: Renal control of acid–base balance

Regarding acid–base balance:

a) Plasma bicarbonate concentration is increased by urinary excretion of hydrogen
b) Renal filtration of hydrogen ions contributes significantly to the maintenance of a normal plasma pH
c) The reabsorption of bicarbonate by the renal tubules is dependent on hydrogen excretion
d) In the collecting tubule, secreted hydrogen will most likely combine with phosphate, not bicarbonate
e) Bicarbonate is freely filtered at the glomerulus

Answer: a,d,e

Short explanation

Hydrogen ions excreted via the kidney are largely secreted rather than filtered (the plasma hydrogen ion concentration is only 36 nmol/L). Bicarbonate reabsorption is dependent on hydrogen secretion but not excretion. As the majority of the filtered bicarbonate is reabsorbed in the early tubular segments, little bicarbonate remains in the distal and collecting tubules to combine with hydrogen. Therefore, in these segments, hydrogen combines with phosphate (which is a buffer that is not reabsorbed).

Long explanation

Bicarbonate ions are freely filtered at the glomerulus, with approximately 4300 mmol filtered per day. Almost all of this filtered bicarbonate is reabsorbed by the proximal tubule (85%), loop of Henle (10%) and the distal tubule and collecting duct. Reabsorption of bicarbonate is dependent on active secretion of hydrogen ions into the tubule fluid. All tubular segments have a hydrogen ATPase pump. However, in the proximal tubule and thick ascending limb of the loop of Henle, this pump is an antiporter that moves hydrogen into the tubule lumen in exchange for sodium reabsorption. Within the tubule lumen, bicarbonate combines with hydrogen to form carbon dioxide and water, both of which diffuse easily into the tubule cells. Once in the cell, in the presence of carbonic anhydrase, carbon dioxide and water combine to form carbonic acid, which subsequently releases a bicarbonate and hydrogen ion. The bicarbonate ion is reabsorbed into the peritubular capillaries while the hydrogen ion is available for active transport out of the cell again. Therefore, bicarbonate reabsorption is dependent on hydrogen secretion but not excretion (as it is recycled).

Each day, a massive amount of volatile and non-volatile acids are produced by the body. Volatile acids are excreted via the lungs, but the kidney excretes approximately 40–80 mmol of non-volatile acids per day as hydrogen ions. As the plasma hydrogen ion concentration is only 36 nmol/L, for a normal glomerular filtration rate of 180 L/day, only 0.684 nmol of hydrogen ions are filtered each day. Therefore, hydrogen ion excretion is largely dependent on secretion. Hydrogen ion secretion is increased by a raised arterial blood carbon dioxide concentration and a high extracellular hydrogen ion concentration. Urinary excretion of hydrogen ions increases the plasma bicarbonate concentration.

Considering the equilibrium equation:

$$CO_2 + H_2O \rightleftharpoons H^+ + HCO_3^-$$

If hydrogen is excreted, the equation is driven to the right, resulting in an increase in plasma bicarbonate excretion. Similarly, if bicarbonate is excreted in the urine, the plasma hydrogen ion concentration will increase.

Power I, Kam P. *Principles of Physiology for the Anaesthetist*. London: Arnold, 2001; pp. 215–19.

MTF Question 28: Liver functional anatomy

Regarding the functional anatomy of the liver, which of the following are correct?

a) There are three lobes of the liver
b) The Couinaud classification describes eight functional segments of the liver
c) The quadrate lobe is segment 1
d) Segment 1 is not visible anteriorly
e) The Bismuth classification divides segment 4 into 4a and 4b

Answer: b,d,e

Short explanation
There are four lobes of the liver: left, right, quadrate and caudate. The caudate lobe is segment 1 in the Couinaud classification.

Long explanation
The liver is the largest organ in the body, weighing 1.5–2 kg. It is divided into the right and left lobes by the attachment of the peritoneum of the falciform ligament. The right lobe is further divided into a quadrate lobe and a caudate lobe. Each lobe of the liver (right and left) can be further subdivided into a number of segments. There are four for each lobe, making eight segments in total.

This classification of liver anatomy is called the Couinaud classification, and it results in eight functionally independent segments. Each segment has its own blood supply, venous drainage and biliary drainage. This means that it is possible to resect a segment entirely without damaging the other segments. The segments are numbered 1 to 8 (the Bismuth classification has a 4a and 4b segment) in a clockwise manner. The numbering starts posteriorly with the caudate lobe (segment 1). It continues anteriorly from the 1 o'clock position. The Bismuth classification is similar to the Couinaud classification but is used more in America.

Further information, with diagrams, is available at www.radiologyassistant.nl/en/ 4375bb8dc241d (accessed 15 March 2012).

MTF Question 29: Neuropathic pain causes

Causes of neuropathic pain include:

a) Carpal tunnel syndrome
b) Persistent immobility
c) Shingles
d) Bipolar depression
e) Multiple sclerosis

Answer: a,c,e

Short explanation

Anything that damages nerves or leads to nerve dysfunction can lead to neuropathic pain. The effects can be mediated peripherally or centrally. Persistent immobility and low mood/depression are 'yellow flags' for chronic back pain.

Long explanation

Pain can be described as nociceptive or neuropathic. Nociceptive pain is a normal response of peripheral nerves to a normal painful stimulus to allow us to respond and move away from that stimulus. When these nerves become damaged, or when dysfunction occurs within the nervous system itself, it can lead to abnormal activation and pain. Often this will resolve as the damaged nerves heal, but because of neuronal plasticity and rewiring of the nervous system persistent chronic (> 3 months) pain may occur.

The cause of neuropathic pain can be almost anything that damages nerves or leads to their dysfunction. Physical damage, infection, ischaemia, metabolic disturbances, immune-mediated reactions and neoplastic disease can all lead to neuropathic pain.

The pain can be divided into central or peripheral pain, depending on the origin of nerve damage or nerve dysfunction. Peripheral pain can originate from the nerve (e.g. carpal tunnel syndrome, phantom limb pain, painful diabetic neuropathy) or dorsal root (e.g. post-herpetic neuralgia). Central pain can originate at the spinal cord level (e.g. spinal cord injury or ischaemia) or in the brain (e.g. post-stroke pain, multiple sclerosis).

Callin, S. Bennett, MI. Assessment of neuropathic pain. *Contin Educ Anaesth Crit Care Pain* 2008; **8**: 210–13. Available online at ceaccp.oxfordjournals.org/content/8/6/210 (accessed 15 March 2012).

MTF Question 30: Sarcomere structure

The sarcomere is the basic contractile unit of skeletal muscle. Which of the following statements are true?

a) Myosin filaments make up the A band
b) The H band is the central area where myosin is not overlapped by actin
c) The thin filament is composed of two myosin filaments wound together with tropomyosin
d) The Z line maintains the spatial relationship of the thin filaments
e) Troponin is composed of three subunits: troponin I, troponin T and troponin C

Answer: a,b,d,e

Short explanation

The thin filament is composed of two actin chains wound together with tropomyosin. The thick myosin filaments contain a head and tail component. The H band contains only myosin filaments. The I band contains only actin filaments.

Long explanation

Skeletal muscle fibres are made up of many myofibrils. The sarcomere is the basic contractile unit, made up of myofibrils. Thin actin filaments and thick myosin filaments are the primary components of the sarcomere and are enclosed by Z lines. A microscopic view of myofibrils demonstrates a striated appearance due to the regular organisation of the thin and thick filaments.

The thin filament consists of two actin chains wound together with tropomyosin. Associated with tropomyosin is the protein complex of troponin, made up of three subunits: troponin I, troponin T and troponin C. The thin filaments maintain their spatial arrangement through their attachment to the Z line. The I band is composed of thin filaments not overlapped by myosin filaments; the I band contains actin only.

Myosin molecules, consisting of a globular head structure and rod-shaped tail, make up the thick filaments. The heads possess actin and ATP binding sites, essential for muscle contraction. The thick filaments form the central A band of the sarcomere. Myosin tails are joined at the central M line. The H band is the region of the myosin filaments that is not overlapped with actin; the H band contains myosin only.

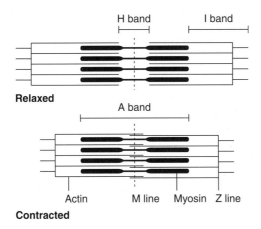

Power I, Kam P. *Principles of Physiology for the Anaesthetist*. London: Arnold, 2001; p. 23–4.

MTF Question 31: Hypertonic saline and ICP

Regarding the use of hypertonic saline to control raised intracranial pressure (ICP):

a) Patients require regular measurement of serum osmolality for therapeutic monitoring
b) The high sodium load makes hypertonic saline more of a potential danger to renal function than mannitol
c) Hypertonic saline should be avoided in hyponatraemic patients
d) Patients receiving hypertonic saline are more haemodynamically stable than those receiving mannitol
e) Current evidence would indicate that hypertonic saline produces a longer-lasting fall in ICP than mannitol osmotherapy

Answer: c,d,e

Short explanation

Hypertonic saline therapy can be satisfactorily monitored with serum sodium measurement and has been found to be less injurious to the kidneys than mannitol.

Long explanation

Mannitol has been the mainstay agent of choice for rapidly managing acutely rising intracranial pressure (ICP) in scenarios such as following severe head injury. In recent years, hypertonic saline has been reintroduced as an alternative therapy. Hypertonic saline was first used for managing traumatic brain injury in 1919.

Like mannitol, hypertonic saline's principal effect is to create an oncotic pressure difference that mobilises water across the blood–brain barrier through osmosis. Hypertonic saline, like mannitol, also has a more rapid effect on improving cerebral perfusion by shrinking erythrocytes and making them more deformable and increasing the calibre of the microcirculation by dehydrating vascular endothelium.

Hypertonic saline is thought to have a number of advantages over mannitol, with less haemodynamic instability, less damage to the kidneys and easier therapeutic monitoring through tracking serum sodium concentration. Hypertonic saline is also less inclined to produce the late rise in ICP sometimes found with mannitol when it is deposited in the brain parenchyma. Hypertonic saline should not be administered to chronically hyponatraemic patients because of the risk of central pontine myelinolysis.

There are no large randomised controlled trials comparing hypertonic saline to mannitol, and the studies available show a lot of heterogeneity. For example, saline concentrations ranging from 3% to 23.4% have been investigated. The available studies indicate that hypertonic saline was a useful rescue therapy if mannitol had failed or could no longer be used and that, when compared to mannitol, hypertonic saline produced a greater size and duration of fall in ICP. No difference in survival between the two agents has been demonstrated.

Brain Trauma Foundation guidelines. 3rd edn, 2007. Available online at www.brain trauma.org/pdf/protected/Guidelines_Management_2007w_bookmarks.pdf (accessed 15 March 2012).

Critically appraised topic 2010, available online at www.bestbets.org/bets/bet.php?id=1977 (accessed 15 March 2012).

White H, Cook D, Venkatesh B. The use of hypertonic saline for treating intracranial hypertension after traumatic brain injury. *Anesth Analg* 2006; **102**: 1836–46. Available online at: www.anesthesiaanalgesia.com/content/102/6/1836.full (accessed 15 March 2012).

MTF Question 32: The management of chronic obstructive pulmonary disease

Regarding the management of chronic obstructive pulmonary disease (COPD):

a) In the absence of significant contraindications, systemic corticosteroids should be prescribed routinely for all patients with exacerbation of COPD admitted to hospital
b) Mucolytics such as carbocisteine have no place in the management of stable COPD
c) More than 15 hours of oxygen a day when on long-term oxygen therapy (LTOT) is undesirable, as outcome deteriorates because of injury by free radicals
d) LTOT improves quality of life but does not prolong survival
e) A patient with an infective exacerbation of COPD should only be given a maximum FiO_2 of 0.3 because of the risk of removing hypoxic drive

Answer: a

Short explanation

Mucolytics are useful for chronic productive cough. LTOT prolongs survival, and 20 hours of oxygen daily has better outcomes than 15 hours but is less well tolerated. Care should be taken when selecting FiO_2 in patients with previous hypercapnic respiratory failure, but most other patients will tolerate a higher FiO_2.

Long explanation

Chronic obstructive pulmonary disease (COPD) is airflow obstruction that is not fully reversible. Airflow limitation does not change over several months, but over the long term usually deteriorates progressively. It is usually caused by smoking, and patients may suffer acute exacerbations, usually related to infections.

NICE published updated guidelines for the management of COPD in 2010. The management plan is comprehensive and covers both chronic state and exacerbations along with guidelines for different levels of severity and different responsiveness to treatment. The first line of managing COPD is to pursue smoking cessation. Initial stages of the guideline are similar to the asthma guideline, with short-acting agents with or without inhaled steroids, with long-acting bronchodilators added in if there are exacerbations or persistent breathlessness. Frequent exacerbations may require vaccination. Chronic productive cough should be treated with a mucolytic.

Respiratory failure may require LTOT. This should be administered for at least 15 hours per day but has even better response if it can be tolerated for 20 hours per day. LTOT has been shown to lengthen survival.

Exacerbation management includes following an algorithm to determine patients requiring hospital admission. All patients admitted to hospital should have inhaled therapy optimised and be started on systemic corticosteroids. Patients with purulent sputum or radiographic evidence of consolidation should be started on antibiotics. In patients who have had a previous episode of hypercapnic respiratory failure, care should be taken to select a low enough FiO_2 to maintain hypoxic respiratory drive. Ideally, these patients should have an accompanying card outlining recommended FiO_2 and target acceptable SpO_2 range. This is a relatively small group of patients and most other patients with exacerbations of COPD will benefit from a higher FiO_2. The oxygen saturation should be measured in all patients with an exacerbation of COPD.

National Institute for Health and Clinical Excellence. *Chronic Obstructive Pulmonary Disease*. NICE Clinical Guideline 101, June 2010. Available online at guidance.nice. org.uk/CG101 (accessed 15 March 2012).

MTF Question 33: Hypertension management

Regarding the pharmacological management of hypertension:

a) An angiotensin-converting enzyme (ACE) inhibitor would be better than a thiazide diuretic as a first-line drug in a 50-year-old female Caucasian patient with hypertension
b) A trial of single agent use should be assessed at 4 weeks
c) Management should target lowering blood pressure to below 140/90 mmHg
d) Severe hypertension (> 180/110 mmHg) usually requires a different group of drugs to the standard hypertension treatment plan
e) Spironolactone would be the best diuretic to add to management of a patient uncontrolled on triple therapy

Answer: a,b,c,e

Short explanation

Hypertension can be managed with the NICE guidelines stepwise plan in the vast majority of cases. This would include the management of severe hypertension.

Long explanation

In the UK, a quarter of the middle-aged and half of the over-65s have hypertension. Hypertension is a resting blood pressure of > 140/90 mmHg, taken on three separate occasions. Treatment should be started if the blood pressure is above 160/100 mmHg or if it is above 140/90 mmHg with raised or cardiovascular risk. The aim is to get the blood pressure below 140/90 mmHg.

NICE published guidelines in 2006, revised in 2011. Step 1 of management usually involves choosing either an ACE inhibitor, a thiazide diuretic or a calcium channel antagonist (A, D and C). An ACE inhibitor is more effective as first-line therapy in younger patients (< 55 years old) and Caucasians. Diuretics or calcium channel antagonists are better in older patients and African/Caribbean patients of any age.

This trial of step 1 is run on for 4 weeks, and if blood pressure is not controlled, the opposite agent is added in. An ACE inhibitor is added to a diuretic (A+D) or calcium channel antagonist (A+C), or vice versa. This constitutes step 2. Ongoing poor control is then managed as step 3 by the addition of the third agent (A+C+D). As part of step 4, if a patient is established on triple therapy, and still not well controlled, they are probably aldosterone sensitive, so spironalactone would be a sensible option.

Most patients with severe hypertension can still be managed with the stepwise plan outlined above. It is rare for a rapid reduction in blood pressure to be required. In very high blood pressure, cerebral autoregulation may be dysfunctional, putting the patient at risk of cerebral infarction if the blood pressure is dropped too rapidly.

National Institute for Health and Clinical Excellence. *Hypertension: Clinical Management of Primary Hypertension in Adults.* NICE Clinical Guideline 127, August 2011. Available online at guidance.nice.org.uk (accessed 15 March 2012).

MTF Question 34: Antigen presentation

Regarding antigen presentation, which of the following statements are correct?

a) Macrophages are capable of presenting foreign particles to B lymphocytes
b) Dendrites, present on antigen-presenting cells, improve interaction with T cells
c) T-cell receptors will recognise antigens presented via the human leucocyte antigen but not the major histocompatibility complex
d) Antigen-presenting cells include epithelial cells
e) Activation of T helper cells stimulates further proliferation of human leucocyte antigen molecules on macrophages

Answer: a,b,d,e

Short explanation
Antigen-presenting cells (APCs) include macrophages, B lymphocytes and dendritic cells. Human leucocyte antigen (HLA) is another term for major histocompatibility complex (MHC) molecules. Macrophages can present antigen to and activate both T and B cells.

Long explanation
Antigen presentation is a process of the immune system by which antigen-presenting cells (APCs) capture antigens and enable recognition by T cells. Antigen-presenting cells include macrophages, B lymphocytes and dendritic cells, as well as non-specific endothelial and epithelial cells. Foreign protein is digested and presented on the cell surface of APCs by major histocompatibility complex (MHC) molecules, also known as human leucocyte antigen (HLA).

Antigens are recognised by a specific T helper cell (Th). Some APCs possess dendrites, long projections which maximise the surface area with which Th cells can interact. Once the Th cell is bound to the antigen–MHC molecule complex, cytokines are released from the macrophage, stimulating Th proliferation. Cytokines are also released from the Th cell, stimulating further production of MHC molecules on macrophages and generating a positive feedback loop.

B cells can be activated through binding of soluble antigen to the B-cell receptor or through the presentation of antigen via an APC.

Harwood NE, Batista FD. Early events in B cell activation. *Annu Rev Immunol* 2010; **28**: 185–210.

Smith T, Pinnock C, Lin T. *Fundamentals of Anaesthesia*, 3rd edn. Cambridge: Cambridge University Press, 2009; p. 245.

MTF Question 35: Endotracheal tubes in children

With regard to the use of endotracheal tubes in children, which of the following statements are true?

a) The glottis is the narrowest part of the airway in children
b) According to Cole's formula the correct size for a 4-year-old would be 5.0 mm internal diameter
c) Nasal endotracheal tubes should be avoided in children under 8 years
d) Uncuffed tubes are not suitable for rapid sequence induction
e) According to Cole's formula the correct size for a 6-year-old would be 6.5 mm internal diameter

Answer: b,c

Short explanation
The cricoid cartilage is the narrowest part of the airway in children. Cole's formula for paediatric tube size is (age/4) + 4. A correctly fitting uncuffed tube provides a secure airway in a child.

Long explanation
There are many differing opinions regarding the correct selection of endotracheal tubes for use in children. However, there are some simple rules that are widely accepted as standard.

The glottis is hexagonal in shape in adults and is the narrowest part of the airway. This means that if an endotracheal tube is passed easily through the vocal cords it should not be tighter-fitting distally, and so the risk of tracheal wall damage is low and the use of a cuff is required to prevent aspiration. In children, the narrowest part of the airway is distal to the glottis, at the level of the cricoid cartilage. This means that a tube that passes smoothly through the vocal cords is likely to be tighter-fitting distally, and so there is no need for a cuff, which could lead to tracheal wall damage. In recent times there has been a move toward using cuffed endotracheal tubes in older children by some. Clinical judgement should be used in individual cases.

There are many guides to the correct size of tube to use in children. Some of these are weight-based and, as the incidence of childhood obesity increases, the standard age-based formula will no doubt become less accurate. The most widely used formula is Cole's formula, which states that tube size should be (age/4) + 4. The size above and below should be directly available when intubating a child. This is important, as there are some ages which, according to the formula, would require a tube size that is not available. For example, a 3-year-old would require a size 4.75 tube. The presence of a leak is often used to decide on exact tube size, particularly in younger children, for whom the standard formula often does not work as well.

Nasal endotracheal tubes should be avoided where possible in children under 8 years, as the adenoids are much larger in this group and any trauma can lead to profuse bleeding.

Al-Shaikh B, Stacey S. *Essentials of Anaesthetic Equipment*, 3rd edn. Edinburgh: Churchill Livingstone, 2007; pp. 68–70.

MTF Question 36: Vitamin K

Regarding vitamin K:

a) It is used as prophylaxis against haemolytic disease of the newborn
b) The body carries no significant stores of vitamin K
c) It is so named because it was discovered after vitamin J (biotin)
d) It is required for the activation of some anticoagulant factors
e) Synthetic oral vitamin K should not be administered to neonates

Answer: d,e

Short explanation
Vitamin K is used in the prophylaxis against haemorrhagic disease of the newborn (quite different from the haemolytic disease). The body stores about 1 week's supply of vitamin K. Vitamin K is so named as it was originally called *Koagulationsvitamin*.

Long explanation
In 1929, Henrik Dam concluded that a group of chickens that had been fed a cholesterol-depleted diet must have also been deficient in a second agent, as the bleeding did not stop when they were fed pure cholesterol. This agent was termed *Koagulationsvitamin* leading to the name vitamin K. Biotin is vitamin B7.

Vitamin K is administered to treat vitamin K deficiency either through inadequate diet or malabsorption, to expedite the reversal of warfarin and in the prophylaxis of the haemorrhagic disease of the newborn. Vitamin K is a fat-soluble vitamin required for the synthesis of six factors in the clotting cascade. These are the coagulant factors II, VII, IX, X and the anticoagulants protein C and protein S. γ-Carboxylation of these factors is carried out by the vitamin K-dependent carboxylase. This reaction subsequently allows calcium binding and the conformational change required to become active. The reaction involves the oxidation of vitamin K. Warfarin works by stopping the reversal of this oxidation.

Two natural forms of vitamin K are found. Vitamin K_1 is found in plant material and vitamin K_2 is synthesised by bacteria in the gut. Bile is required for absorption of vitamin K in the gut. The body stores about 1 week's supply of vitamin K. Menadiol, a third synthesised form of vitamin K (K_3), is water-soluble and therefore can be absorbed in conditions in which bile secretion is low. It is not recommended for use in neonates as it may produce haemolysis.

Prophylaxis against haemorrhagic disease of the newborn is usually given at birth as an injection of the naturally occurring fat-soluble phytomenadione. Haemorrhagic disease of the newborn is caused by a relative vitamin K deficiency. Haemolytic disease of the newborn is usually due to an immunologically mediated reaction in which antibodies (usually IgG) from the maternal circulation cross the placenta and attack the neonate's erythrocytes.

Bennett P N, Brown M J. *Clinical Pharmacology*, 10th edn. Edinburgh: Churchill Livingstone Elsevier, 2008; pp. 514–15.

MTF Question 37: Propofol

Which of the following statements about propofol are true?

a) Propofol is contraindicated in patients with an allergy to eggs
b) Excitatory movements seen on induction with propofol are due to epileptiform EEG activity
c) Propofol is 75% protein-bound in plasma

d) Propofol causes more cardiovascular changes than thiopental when used in equi-analgesic doses

e) Pain on injection of propofol can be reduced by injecting into a fast-flowing intravenous drip

Answer: d,e

Short explanation
The egg phosphatide used as an emulsifying agent in propofol is denatured by the manufacturing process. No epileptiform EEG changes are seen with propofol. Propofol is 98% protein-bound.

Long explanation
Propofol (2,6-di-isopropyl phenol) is an alkylated phenol. It is presented as a white emulsion at concentrations of 1% or 2% with soya bean oil (10%), purified egg phosphatide (1.2%) and glycerol (2.25%); the solution has a pH of 6.5–8.0 and is stable at room temperature and not light-sensitive. The soya bean oil and egg components are denatured by processing and there is no evidence that propofol should be avoided in patients with allergies to eggs or soya.

Its pKa is 11 and so it is almost entirely un-ionised in solution; in the plasma it is 98% protein-bound. It causes dose-dependent depression of cortical activity, with the EEG showing alpha waves followed by delta waves as anaesthesia deepens. Excitatory movements are seen relatively commonly although there are no epileptiform features on the EEG; indeed, propofol has good anticonvulsant activity and can be used to treat status epilepticus.

Propofol causes a reduction in systemic vascular resistance and central venous pressure by vasodilation, and also reduces myocardial contractility. This reduces blood pressure, and the heart rate is usually unchanged. These cardiovascular effects are more pronounced than those produced by barbiturates at equi-anaesthetic doses. More respiratory depression is seen with propofol than with barbiturates (apnoea is universal) and propofol supresses the response to laryngoscopy more than thiopental does.

One of the problems with propofol is pain on injection. This is increased by injection into a small vein, rapid injection, lower temperature of the propofol and the use of an IV carrier infusion to dilute the propofol as it enters the vein. Adding 2 mL of 1% lidocaine to a 20 mL syringe of propofol or giving the same dose prior to propofol administration is effective at attenuating this symptom.

Pandit J. Intravenous anaesthetic agents. *Anaesth Intens Care Med* 2007; **9** (4): 154–9.
Smith T, Pinnock C, Lin T. *Fundamentals of Anaesthesia*, 3rd edn. Cambridge: Cambridge University Press, 2009.

MTF Question 38: Impedance

Which of the following statements correctly describe the principles of impedance?

a) The unit of impedance is the same as that of resistance
b) Impedance is given the symbol Ω
c) Skin impedance is lower when the skin is moist
d) Defibrillation may be more effective during inspiration than expiration
e) Impedance is inversely proportional to current frequency

Answer: a,c

Short explanation
Impedance is given the symbol Z. Thoracic impedance is higher during inspiration, suggesting that defibrillation may be more effective during expiration. Impedance

defines the resistance of a system when the resistance is dependent on current frequency; it is not itself frequency-dependent.

Long explanation

A capacitor allows the transmission of alternating current within a circuit. As the frequency of the current increases, the current passes through the circuit more easily, i.e. the resistance of the capacitor falls with increasing current frequency. In contrast, the resistance of an inductor rises as the frequency of the current increases.

Where the resistance of a circuit is dependent on the frequency of the current through it, the term impedance is used. The unit of impedance is therefore the same as that of resistance (the ohm), but the symbol Z is used to differentiate it from the symbol used for resistance (Ω).

Impedance is a term that is commonly used in the world of electrophysiology and biomechanical engineering. You are more likely to get an electric shock when you have wet hands because the impedance of your skin is lower than when it is dry. Thoracic impedance increases during inspiration. When applying electric current to the chest during defibrillation, less energy may reach the heart during the inspiratory phase than during the expiratory phase because of this phenomenon, thereby decreasing the possible success of defibrillation. This is one of the reasons why defibrillation is attempted during the expiratory phase of mechanical ventilation.

Davis PD, Kenny GNC. *Basic Physics and Measurement in Anaesthesia*, 5th edn. Oxford: Butterworth–Heinemann, 2003; pp. 149–64.

Ewy GA, Hellman DA, McClung S, Taren D. Influence of ventilation phase on transthoracic impedance and defibrillation effectiveness. *Crit Care Med* 1980; **8**: 164–6.

MTF Question 39: Sedation in children and young people

Regarding sedation in children and young adults:

a) Fasting is not required for minimal sedation
b) Intravenous propofol, with or without fentanyl or intravenous ketamine, is recommended for deep sedation for painful procedures
c) Intravenous midazolam with fentanyl is recommended for upper gastrointestinal endoscopy
d) Opioids are not recommended for non-painful procedures
e) Chloral hydrate has no place in the sedation of children

Answer: a,b,d

Short explanation

Midazolam without fentanyl is recommended for upper gastrointestinal endoscopy. Chloral hydrate is indicated in children under 15 kg for sedation for non-painful procedures.

Long explanation

In 2010 the National Institute for Health and Clinical Excellence (NICE) released guidelines for sedation in children and young people. Most of the guideline is common sense and corresponds with general advice released by AAGBI regarding sedation in adults.

Potentially painful procedures should be assessed and a judgement made about whether minimal, moderate or deep sedation is required. NICE states that fasting is not required for minimal sedation and recommends oral or intranasal midazolam or sedation with nitrous oxide (up to 50%). Recommendations for moderate sedation are to use nitrous oxide or intravenous midazolam with or without fentanyl. Deep sedation should be with propofol, with or without fentanyl or intravenous ketamine.

For sedation for painless procedures such as diagnostic imaging, the guidelines recommend chloral hydrate for children under 15 kg, propofol or sevoflurane. Ketamine or opioids should not routinely be used for painless procedure sedation.

Intravenous midazolam is recommended for both upper and lower gastrointestinal endoscopy. Additional fentanyl may also be needed for lower gastrointestinal endoscopy. Nitrous oxide or midazolam is recommended for dental procedures if local anaesthesia is not tolerated. If these techniques are inadequate, the child should be referred to a specialist team for other sedative techniques.

National Institute for Health and Clinical Excellence. *Sedation in Children and Young People: Sedation for Diagnostic and Therapeutic Procedures in Children and Young people.* NICE Clinical Guideline 112, December 2010. Available online at guidance.nice.org. uk/CG112 (accessed 15 March 2012).

MTF Question 40: Draw-over vaporisers

Draw-over vaporisers:

a) Are driven by downstream negative pressure
b) Have a high resistance to flow
c) Are often used 'in the field' because of their portability
d) Require an external cylinder gas supply
e) Are positioned inside the breathing system

Answer: a,c,e

Short explanation
Draw-over vaporisers are placed inside the breathing circuit and therefore must have a very low resistance to flow to avoid additional resistance to the patient's breathing.

Long explanation
Examples of draw-over vaporisers include the Goldman vaporiser, the Oxford miniature vaporiser (OMV) and the Epstein MacIntosh vaporiser (EMV). They are placed inside the breathing system and rely on a negative pressure downstream from the vaporiser to create the flow required to entrain the agent. This negative pressure is generated either by the patient's own inspiration or by a self-inflating bag. For this reason, draw-over vaporisers must have a low resistance to flow.

Compared to plenum vaporisers, draw-over vaporisers are simpler, more lightweight, smaller and less expensive. They do not require an external cylinder gas supply and are therefore of use 'in the field', when portability is desired. The triservice apparatus, used by the military, incorporates two OMVs.

The major disadvantage of draw-over vaporisers is their inaccuracy. This is because it is not possible to calibrate for the large range of tidal volumes created by the patient/ self-inflating bag. For this reason, they are not generally used in Western hospitals, and are reserved for out-of-hospital, 'in-the-field' use, where portability is required.

Al-Shaikh B, Stacey S. *Essentials of Anaesthetic Equipment*, 2nd edn. Edinburgh: Churchill Livingstone, 2002.
Davis PD, Kenny GNC. *Basic Physics and Measurement in Anaesthesia*, 5th edn. Oxford: Butterworth–Heinemann, 2003.

MTF Question 41: Tec 6 vaporiser

The Tec Mk 6 vaporiser:

a) Is an example of a plenum vaporiser
b) Has a chamber operating temperature of 29 °C
c) Is made of copper

d) Has a warm-up time of 30 seconds

e) Requires an external power supply

Answer: a,c,e

Short explanation

The desflurane vaporiser is a plenum vaporiser. However, it is unique in that it operates at a specific temperature of 39 °C and a pressure of 2 atmospheres (the others all operate at atmospheric pressure and temperature). It takes 5–10 minutes to warm up to the correct temperature.

Long explanation

Desflurane has a saturated vapour pressure of 664 mmHg at 20 °C and a boiling point of 22.6 °C. This is lower than the other volatile agents, and it therefore requires a specific vaporiser for its use.

The Tec Mk 6 vaporiser has been designed specifically for desflurane. The vaporisation chamber is heated to 39 °C with a pressure of 2 atmospheres. It therefore needs an external power supply, and it also has a 9 V battery in case of mains failure. After switching the vaporiser on, it takes 5–10 minutes to warm up to the correct temperature. It will not operate until the vaporisation chamber has reached 39 °C.

Unlike the other plenum vaporisers, the Tec Mk 6 vaporiser is designed so that the fresh gas flow does not enter the chamber. The desflurane vapour is added to the fresh gas flow as it leaves the vaporiser.

When the percentage control dial on the top of the vaporiser is adjusted by the operator, a variable flow restriction is applied to desflurane vapour flow. The desflurane vapour is then added to the fresh gas flow output. However, this is not the whole story. What would happen if we increased or decreased the fresh gas flow? A fixed flow of desflurane vapour would result in very different inspired concentrations if it was mixed with a fresh gas flow of 15 L/min compared to a fresh gas flow of 300 mL/min. To overcome this, the vaporiser incorporates a differential pressure transducer.

As the fresh gas flow goes through the vaporiser (but not the chamber) it flows through a fixed restriction, which alters the flow (and therefore pressure) of the gas flowing through it. The differential pressure transducer senses the pressure difference between the fresh gas flow at the fixed restriction and the desflurane pressure upstream of the pressure regulating valve. It then adjusts an electronic valve at the outlet of the vaporising chamber to ensure that the pressure of the desflurane upstream of the control valve equals the pressure of fresh gas flow at the fixed restriction. This means that at varying flow rates, the concentration of desflurane in the inspired gases is maintained at the desired percentage set by the operator. Genius!

Al-Shaikh B, Stacey S. *Essentials of Anaesthetic Equipment*, 2nd edn. Edinburgh: Churchill Livingstone, 2002.

Davis PD, Kenny GNC. *Basic Physics and Measurement in Anaesthesia*, 5th edn. Oxford: Butterworth–Heinemann, 2003.

MTF Question 42: Drug uptake

Which of the following statements about drug uptake are true?

a) Hepatic first-pass metabolism of propranolol is influenced by the degree of protein binding

b) Rectal administration of drugs improves absorption compared to oral administration

c) Vecuronium is ionised in the stomach and largely absorbed in the small intestine

d) Where hepatic metabolic capacity for a drug is high, first-pass metabolism is dependent on hepatic blood flow

e) Nasal administration has the advantage of rapid onset of action

Answers: d,e

Short explanation

The metabolic capacity for propranolol is high, so the main influence on its metabolism is hepatic blood flow. Protein binding influences the metabolism of drugs with a lower metabolic capacity. Absorption from the rectum is often worse than oral absorption. Vecuronium is permanently ionised and not absorbed from the gut.

Long explanation

After oral administration drugs must cross the gut mucosa into the portal circulation and pass through the liver before entering the systemic circulation. Only un-ionised molecules can cross the mucosal barrier, meaning that weakly acidic drugs (e.g. aspirin) begin to be absorbed in the acidic environment of the stomach while weakly basic drugs only begin to be absorbed in the small intestine. Drugs that are permanently ionised (e.g. the non-depolarising muscle relaxants) are not absorbed from the gut at all.

Metabolism occurring in the gut wall (e.g. GTN) or in the liver is called 'first-pass' metabolism and reduces the amount of drug that reaches its effect site. The extraction ratio is the fraction of the total oral dose that is removed before reaching the systemic circulation, and it is dependent on hepatic blood flow, uptake of drug into the hepatocyte and hepatocellular metabolic capacity for the drug.

Propranolol is an example of a drug with a high metabolic capacity, and any drug entering the hepatocyte is quickly broken down. This maintains a concentration gradient favouring the dissociation of the drug from protein binding sites, and means that overall hepatic metabolism is mainly related to hepatic blood flow. Phenytoin, however, has a much lower hepatic metabolic capacity and hence remains bound to protein. In this case the degree of protein binding (as affected by other drugs competing for binding sites) influences entry to the hepatocyte more than the hepatic blood flow and becomes the main determinant of the extraction ratio.

Rectal, sublingual and nasal routes have the advantage of bypassing the portal circulation and avoiding first-pass metabolism. The sublingual and nasal routes also give a rapid onset of action, but absorption from the rectal route is slow and can be incomplete.

Peck T, Hill S, Williams M. *Pharmacology for Anaesthesia and Intensive Care*, 3rd edn. Cambridge: Cambridge University Press, 2008.

MTF Question 43: Needles and cannulae

Which of the following statements correctly describes the structure of epidural equipment?

a) The bevel of the epidural needle is angled at 30° to the shaft

b) The bevel of the Tuohy needle is known as a Crawford point

c) The paediatric Tuohy needle has markings in 0.5 cm increments

d) The epidural catheter is made of PTFE

e) Fluid does not leave through the tip of the epidural catheter; it only exits through side ports

Answer: c,e

Short explanation

The bevel of the Tuohy needle is angled at 20° to the shaft of the needle and is known as a Huber point. The epidural catheter is made of nylon or Teflon. The design of the distal end of the epidural catheter is as described to avert vascular or dural puncture.

Long explanation

Epidural needles are used to identify and cannulate the epidural space. The commonest needle used to perform this procedure in the UK is the Tuohy needle, which has particular design features making it both safe and easy to use. The commonest size of Tuohy needle is 16 or 18 gauge, and 10 cm in length. The shaft of this needle is 8 cm long, having markings in 1 cm increments, allowing the identification of the distance from the skin to the epidural space. Needles of 15 cm are available for those with an adverse body mass index.

An introducer prevents coring of tissue on insertion of the needle, which might result in blockage. The tip of the needle has a bevel known as a Huber point, which is angled obliquely at 20° to the shaft of the needle. This blunt, obliquely angled tip allows identification of the epidural space using a loss of resistance technique, where a sharp needle would pass through the ligaments without a change in palpable feedback to the operator.

Paediatric Tuohy needles are available. These 19 gauge, 5 cm long needles have markings in 0.5 cm increments.

The adult epidural catheter is 90 cm long and is made of nylon or Teflon. The distal tip of the catheter is rounded and closed, preventing fluid from leaving the catheter by this route. Fluid instead leaves from two or more side ports at the distal end of the catheter. This design reduces the risk of vascular or dural puncture.

Al-Shaikh B, Stacey S. *Essentials of Anaesthetic Equipment*, 2nd edn. Edinburgh: Churchill Livingstone, 2002; pp. 151–4.

MTF Question 44: Adjustable pressure-limiting (APL) valves

Which of the following are true regarding the adjustable pressure-limiting (APL) valve?

a) The APL valve allows positive-pressure ventilation when completely unscrewed
b) During periods of high flow (e.g. at peak inspiration), it is possible to entrain room air through the APL valve during spontaneous respiration
c) Modern APL valves incorporate a secondary overpressure relief valve, which prevents the circuit pressure rising above 60 cmH_2O
d) The overpressure relief valve is redundant in modern breathing circuits, as the distensible reservoir bag prevents excessive pressure rises
e) The APL valve will produce positive end-expiratory pressure (PEEP)

Answers: c,e

Short explanation

When unscrewed, the APL will open at 1.5 cmH_2O, preventing application of significant positive pressure to the patient's lungs. A functional APL will not allow entrainment of room air. Modern reservoir bags are less compliant than older latex ones, and so the relief valve remains an important safety feature.

Long explanation

The APL valve consists of a lightweight disc resting on a knife-edge circular seating which results in a minimal surface contact area (this reduces the chance of sticking with condensation). A spring is mounted to the top, the tension of which is adjusted by the user by turning a screw. When the circuit has negative pressure applied (e.g. on patient inspiration) the valve will close, and no entrainment of room air should be possible. When the screw is completely loosened, the spring is slack, and the valve will open when a pressure of around 1.5 cmH$_2$O is applied to it, allowing minimal resistance to expiration in a spontaneously breathing patient. This, however, prevents the use of positive-pressure ventilation, as the rise in pressure is lost through the valve.

When the valve is fully screwed down, it will allow pressure to build up in the circuit. To prevent this reaching a dangerous level, a safety overpressure release valve is normally incorporated in modern APL valves. This will start to open at a pressure of 30 cmH$_2$O, and will be fully open at a pressure of 60 cmH$_2$O, when it will allow gas to escape at a rate of 50 L/min.

The reservoir bag was traditionally made of natural latex, until this was removed because of the increasing rate of latex allergy. The latex bags were very compliant, and if excess gas entered the circuit they would distend, rather than allowing the pressure in the circuit to rise, and would rupture before potentially injurious pressures occurred. However, the overpressure relief valve was still important in case this should fail – for instance, if the bag was trapped under the operating table. Modern bags do not have the same elasticity, and so are less compliant, therefore making the overpressure valve even more important.

The APL valve will always produce a small resistance to expiration, even when maximally loosened, producing low levels of PEEP. This resistance increases as the valve is tightened, and valves have been designed to allow titratable, measurable levels of PEEP through the valve.

Davey A, Diba A. Breathing systems and their components. In: *Ward's Anaesthetic Equipment*, 5th edn. Philadephia, PA: Saunders, 2005; pp. 131–63.

MTF Question 45: Iron absorption

Iron absorption:

a) Primarily occurs in the terminal ileum
b) Is independent of total body stores
c) Is extremely efficient
d) Occurs via active transport
e) Binds apoferritin once inside intestinal cells

Answers: d,e

Short explanation

Iron absorption occurs in the duodenum and jejunum, depending on total body iron stores. Only a small percentage of total dietary iron is actually absorbed as either haem or free iron.

Long explanation

Dietary iron is ingested either as free iron or as iron bound to haem molecules. Haem-bound iron is mainly sourced from red meat. Iron absorption is not very efficient. Of the total ingested, we only absorb 5–25%, the amount absorbed being dependent on total body stores. As we cannot metabolise iron we depend on slow losses through bleeding, menstruation, cell sloughing etc. to keep the levels within normal range, and only absorb what we need.

Iron overload can have serious clinical implications, as seen in haemochromatosis. This is a disease of iron overload that can lead to effects such as cardiomyopathy, diabetes mellitus, liver cirrhosis and hepatocellular carcinoma.

The absorption of iron primarily occurs across the duodenal and jejunal mucosa. Free iron is absorbed by active transport once it has bound to a specific receptor on the apical membrane of the intestinal cell. The expression of this receptor is linked to the total body iron stores. Iron bound to haem enters via pinocytosis and is released as free iron when the haem molecule is broken down.

Inside the cell the free iron binds apoferritin to form ferritin. Ferritin is the intracellular iron storage molecule. If required, free iron is released into the plasma across the basement membrane. Here it binds a β-globulin transport molecule known as transferrin. Transferrin production is also linked to total body iron stores

Smith T, Pinnock C, Lin T. *Fundamentals of Anaesthesia*, 3rd edn. Cambridge: Cambridge University Press, 2009; p. 446.

MTF Question 46: Peak flow

Regarding the measurement of peak expiratory flow rate:

a) Results depend on patient effort
b) It may be measured with a pneumotachograph
c) It is the maximal rate of airflow during passive expiration
d) Normal values in females are 350–600 mL/min
e) Normal values in males are 450–700 L/min

Answer: a,b,e

Short explanation

Peak expiratory flow rate is the maximal rate of airflow during forced expiration. It is therefore very dependent on patient effort. It may be measured by a pneumotachograph. Normal values are 250–500 L/min for women and 450–700 L/min for men.

Long explanation

Peak expiratory flow rate is the maximal rate of airflow during forced expiration. It is therefore very dependent on patient effort. Measurements are taken three times and the best of the three results is used.

Peak expiratory flow rate is usually measured by a peak flowmeter, but it may also be measured by a pneumotachograph or flow–volume loops. The Wright peak flowmeter is a constant-pressure, variable-orifice device. It can measure flow rates of up to 1000 L/min. It is a very simple, hand-held device and is commonly used in clinical practice. The pneumotachograph is a variable-pressure, constant-orifice device. It is usually used for research purposes and in cardiopulmonary exercise testing. Flow–volume loops are graphs representing airflows at different lung volumes. They can help distinguish between obstructive and restrictive airways disease.

Normal values of peak expiratory flow rate depend on sex and age, but are typically in the range of 250–500 L/min for women and 450–700 L/min for men. Note that the units of measurement are L/min. Values are reduced in obstructive airways disease. The trend in peak flow measurements can be useful in determining the severity of an acute episode, and also in evaluating the response to treatments.

Yentis S, Hirsch N, Smith G. *Anaesthesia and Intensive Care A–Z: an Encyclopaedia of Principles and Practice*, 3rd edn. Edinburgh: Butterworth–Heinemann, 2004; pp. 211, 404, 419.

MTF Question 47: Carcinoid syndrome

In the perioperative management of a patient having surgery for carcinoid syndrome:

a) Thiopental would be a good choice of induction agent
b) Morphine would be a good choice of narcotic analgesic
c) Intraoperative hypotension may be improved by the administration of octreotide

d) Regional anaestheisa avoids most of the major complications caused by general anaesthesia

e) Ondansetron is the agent of choice to prevent postoperative nausea and vomiting

Answer: c,e

Short explanation
Thiopental and morphine may cause decompensation in carcinoid syndrome, as they may produce histamine release. Regional anaesthesia is controversial, as it may cause severe hypotension that is difficult to treat.

Long explanation
Carcinoid tumours are neuroendocrine neoplasias usually originating from entero-chromaffin cells. Ninety per cent are found in the gastrointestinal tract, although they may be found in many other sites such as the bronchus or gonads. They are usually indolent and the patient is asymptomatic. If symptoms do occur they commonly present with abdominal pain, diarrhoea, gastrointestinal obstruction and bleeding, or from the mechanical effects of tumours. They commonly secrete serotonin, but this is metabol-ised on first pass through the liver. Treatment options for symptomatic patients are excision, chemotherapy, or biotherapy with octreotide and interferon.

Fifteen per cent of patients with carcinoid tumours suffer from carcinoid syndrome. Neuropeptides and amines are secreted into the systemic circulation, usually because of lung or liver metastases. The patient is symptomatic of neuropeptides either because they are released without going through the portal circulation or because they are at such a high level that they overwhelm the liver's capacity to metabolise them all. Carcinoid tumours may secrete serotonin, histamine, bradykinin, tachykinin, motilin, substance P, kallikrein, prostaglandins, catecholamines and other bio-active com-pounds. Common symptoms include hypo- or hypertension, flushing, bronchocon-striction, diarrhoea and carcinoid heart disease. In carcinoid heart disease, the patient develops thickened valves and chordae resulting in tricuspid and pulmonary regur-gitation and pulmonary stenosis (and more rarely mitral and aortic insufficiency). Also pericarditis or myocardial metastases may occur.

Treatment for carcinoid syndrome may include surgical resection or debulking, but is also pharmacological. Cardiopulmonary effects are managed acutely with octreotide intravenously, and chronically with long-acting depot somatostatin analogues such as lanreotide. Drugs releasing histamine (thiopental, suxamethonium, atracurium, mor-phine) should be avoided, as should catecholamines if at all possible.

Regional anaesthesia is controversial because of hypotension. The mainstay treat-ment is intravenous octreotide for both prophylaxis and intraoperative crises such as bronchospasm or low blood pressure. If the tumour is gastric, give prophylactic antihist-amines. Vasoactive drugs may produce crises. A test dose is advisable. Historically, ketanserin, methysergide, cyproheptadine and aprotonin were used. Postoperatively, ensure effective analgesia, continue octreotide, and give ondansetron for PONV.

Dierdorf SF. Carcinoid tumour and carcinoid syndrome. *Curr Opin Anaesthesiol* 2003; **16**: 343–7.

MTF Question 48: Thyroid hormones

Regarding thyroid hormone secretion and thyroid-stimulating hormone (TSH):

a) TSH increases the uptake of thyroid hormones by thyroglobulin

b) Thyroxine-binding globulin (TBG) has the greatest capacity to bind thyroxine compared with other plasma proteins

c) Reduced protein binding results in increased free hormone

d) Cold increases circulating TSH levels
e) Glucocorticoids stimulate TSH secretion

Answer: d

Short explanation

TSH releases the hormones from thyroglobulin. Albumin has the greatest capacity for thyroxine. Free hormone levels are maintained constant irrespective of protein binding levels. Glucocorticoids inhibit TSH secretion.

Long explanation

Thyroid hormones are synthesised in the thyroid gland, regulated by thyroid-stimulating hormone (TSH) and thyrotrophin-releasing hormone (TRH). Tri-iodothyronine (T_3) and tetra-iodothyronine (thyroxine, T_4) are produced from tyrosine derived from thyroglobulin and combined with iodine. Although T_4 is produced in the majority, T_3 has five times the activity of T_4.

Once produced, these hormones are bound to thyroglobulin until ready for secretion. Secretion of TSH occurs from the anterior pituitary under the control of TRH from the hypothalamus. The TSH releases T_3 and T_4 from thyroglobulin and into the bloodstream. TSH also increases the size and number of the thyroid gland cells, potentially leading to goitre formation if unchecked. TSH increases hormone production while releasing that already produced. It also increases iodide binding, thyroglobulin release into the colloid of the thyroid gland and endocytosis of colloid by the thyroid cells.

Once in the bloodstream these hormones are 99% protein-bound. There are several different plasma proteins to which thyroxine can bind, including albumin, thyroxine-binding prealbumin (TBPA) and thyroxine-binding globulin (TBG). Of these, albumin has the greatest capacity to bind thyroxine but TBG has the greatest affinity. Should the levels of protein fall, the proportion of free unbound thyroxine remains relatively constant. It is the free unbound portion that provides negative feedback to the anterior pituitary and hypothalamus to regulate TSH levels. As well as negative feedback, other factors alter thyroxine production. Stress, blood glucose and basal metabolic rate can alter TRH release. Stress has an inhibitory effect. Temperature affects hormone production: warmth decreases production and cold increases it. Glucocorticoids, like dopamine and somatostatin, inhibit TSH secretion.

Smith T, Pinnock C, Lin T. *Fundamentals of Anaesthesia*, 3rd edn. Cambridge: Cambridge University Press, 2009; p. 474.

MTF Question 49: Sickle cell disease

Regarding sickle cell disease, which of the following statements are true?

a) Sickle cell disease is due to a single DNA base change on the β-globin chain, rendering the molecule more hydrophilic
b) The affinity of dissolved sickle haemoglobin for oxygen is the same as that of normal haemoglobin
c) The degree of precipitation of sickle haemoglobin is dependent on the concentration of deoxygenated haemoglobin.
d) A patient with sickle cell disease may also have normal haemoglobin A
e) Sickle haemoglobin precipitates at a PO_2 of 3–4 kPa

Answer: b,c

Short explanation

A single DNA base change results in the synthesis of abnormal, hydrophobic haemoglobin. This haemoglobin can precipitate and polymerise at a PO_2 of 5–6 kPa. The overall affinity of haemoglobin S for oxygen is reduced due to polymerisation, but the affinity of dissolved haemoglobin S is comparable to that of haemoglobin A. Sickle cell disease is the homozygous condition, in which only haemoglobin S is produced.

Long explanation

Sickle cell disease is an autosomal dominant haemoglobinopathy, where a mutation results in the synthesis of abnormal haemoglobin. It is due to a single DNA base change (adenine for thymine) resulting in an amino acid substitution of valine for glutamic acid on the β chain. As valine is a hydrophobic amino acid, and glutamic acid hydrophilic, the deoxygenated haemoglobin molecule is less soluble, and susceptible to precipitation and polymerisation. Dissolved sickle haemoglobin (HbS) has the same affinity for oxygen as haemoglobin A. However, overall affinity is reduced as some of the HbS will be polymerised.

Heterozygotes for the sickle mutation synthesise both normal HbA and abnormal HbS. This condition is classified as sickle cell trait and is associated with normal development, exercise tolerance and life expectancy.

The homozygous condition produces only abnormal haemoglobin. Presenting features include haemolysis and anaemia, impaired tissue perfusion, end-organ dysfunction and acute vascular occlusion. Sickling of red blood cells is dependent on a number of factors including hypothermia, infection, dehydration and hypoxaemia. As mentioned above, HbS can polymerise and precipitate within red blood cells, causing distortion and increased rigidity. Sickled cells cause an increase in blood viscosity, leading to impaired blood flow and occlusion of vessels. Ultimately, organ infarction may occur. Regarding hypoxaemia, HbS will precipitate at a PO_2 of 5–6 kPa. Within this range falls the PO_2 of venous blood. Therefore, homozygotes with only abnormal haemoglobin are constantly sickling. Heterozygotes experience sickling at a much lower PO_2, 2.5–4 kPa.

Diagnosis is by detection of HbS. The commonly used Sickledex test involves the addition of a reagent to the blood and observation for turbidity. If even a small amount of HbS is present, the test will be positive. Therefore it cannot be used to distinguish between patients with sickle cell trait and those with the homozygous disease.

Smith T, Pinnock C, Lin T. *Fundamentals of Anaesthesia*, 3rd edn. Cambridge: Cambridge University Press, 2009; pp. 234–5.
Yentis S, Hirsch N, Smith G. *Anaesthesia and Intensive Care A–Z: an Encyclopaedia of Principles and Practice*, 3rd edn. Edinburgh: Butterworth–Heinemann, 2004; pp. 471–2.

MTF Question 50: Measurement of gas and vapour concentrations

Which of the following are true regarding the measurement of gas and vapour concentrations?

a) The presence of water vapour in a sample will increase the concentration of other gases
b) Saturated vapour pressure is needed to correct for water vapour
c) Barometric pressure is needed to correct for water vapour
d) Water vapour can be removed by silica gel
e) Water vapour is removed by modern gas analysers

Answer: b,c,d,e

Short explanation

Water vapour reduces the concentration of other gases in a mixture. Both the saturated vapour pressure and barometric pressure are needed to correct for the presence of water vapour. Water vapour can be removed by silica gel. Many modern gas analysers remove water vapour from gases before they are analysed.

Long explanation

The presence of water vapour in a mixture of dry gases can affect the accuracy of concentration measurements. The partial pressure of each gas component in a mixture will be reduced because of the partial pressure of the water vapour. A correction can be made for humidified gases using the partial pressure of the humidified gas, the barometric pressure and the saturated vapour pressure of water at a given temperature.

$$\text{Concentration} = \frac{\text{Partial pressure (humidified at } 37\,^\circ\text{C)}}{\text{Barometric pressure} - \text{SVP of water at } 37\,^\circ\text{C}}$$

As an alternative to the correction, the humidified gases can be dried before analysis. This is the case in many modern gas analysers. One such method is by passing the gases through a drying agent such as silica gel.

Davies PD, Kenny GNC. *Basic Physics and Measurement in Anaesthesia*, 5th edn. Oxford: Butterworth–Heinemann, 2003; p. 209.

MTF Question 51: Suxamethonium

Regarding suxamethonium:

a) It is a dicholine ester of succinic acid
b) When presented as the bromide salt it is supplied as a powder and needs to be dissolved in sterile water before use
c) It is made up of two molecules of acetylcholine (ACh) joined via their hydroxyl groups
d) It can be presented as the fluoride salt
e) When presented as the chloride salt it is supplied as a 100 mg/mL solution

Answer: a,b

Short explanation

Suxamethonium is made up of two molecules of ACh joined via their acetyl groups. It can be presented as the chloride, bromide or iodide salt. The chloride salt is a solution of 50 mg/mL.

Long explanation

Suxamethonium is currently the only available depolarising muscle relaxant in clinical practice. Decamethonium used to be available but is now only used for research purposes. The basic structure of suxamethonium is two molecules of acetylcholine (ACh) linked via their acetyl groups.

When presented as the chloride salt it is a solution of concentration 50 mg/mL. It must be kept refrigerated at around 4 °C to prevent degradation. The bromide and iodide salts are presented as powder, which must be reconstituted with sterile water before use. The powder is more stable and has a longer shelf life, which makes it more suitable for warmer climates. All solutions of suxamethonium are destroyed by alkali and should not be mixed with thiopental. The pH of the solutions is around 4.

Kestin I. Suxamethonium. *Update in Anaesthesia* 1992; **1**: article 7. Available online at www.nda.ox.ac.uk/wfsa/html/u01/u01_010.htm (accessed 15 March 2012).
Peck T, Hill S, Williams M. *Pharmacology for Anaesthesia and Intensive Care*, 3rd edn. Cambridge: Cambridge University Press, 2008; pp. 179–84.

MTF Question 52: Monitoring the depth of anaesthesia

Regarding the bispectral index (BIS) value scale, which of the following are true?

a) A value of 80 represents an awake patient
b) A value of 40–60 is recommended for general anaesthesia
c) Patient temperature has no effect on the BIS value
d) Cerebral ischaemia reduces the BIS value
e) A value of zero indicates a flatline EEG

Answer: b,d,e

Short explanation
The BIS value scale is a dimensionless scale between zero and 100. A value of 100 represents an awake patient. Both hypothermia and global cerebral ischaemia reduce the BIS value.

Long explanation
BIS (bispectral index) is used in the statistical analysis of components of the electro-encephalogram (EEG). A linear and dimensionless scale is produced from zero (no EEG activity) to 100 (an awake patient). Values of 40–60 are recommended for general anaesthesia; at 60 patients begin to return to consciousness. Values of 65–85 are recommended for sedation, although sedation with ketamine cannot be monitored in this manner as it causes an increase in EEG activity. Both hypothermia and global cerebral ischaemia will cause a reduction in BIS value because both cause a slowing of brain processing and EEG activity.

Al Shaikh B, Stacey S. *Essentials of Anaesthetic Equipment*, 3rd edn. Edinburgh: Churchill Livingstone, 2007; pp. 151–3.

MTF Question 53: Insulin and the insulin receptor

Regarding insulin and the insulin receptor:

a) Insulin has a tertiary protein structure
b) Insulin is produced from preproinsulin in the endoplasmic reticulum
c) The insulin receptor has two α and two β subunits.
d) Receptor binding results in production of cell membrane transporters
e) The insulin receptor activates adenylyl cyclase via a second-messenger system

Answer: b,c

Short explanation
Insulin has a secondary protein structure which activates its second-messenger system via tyrosine kinase. Binding results in cell membrane transporters, already stored in cell vesicles, being incorporated into the cell membrane.

Long explanation
Insulin is produced in the islets of Langerhans cells that sit between the acini and ducts of the pancreatic lobules. There are several different types of islet cells, and insulin is produced by the β cells, contributing up to 75% of the islets' secretions.

Insulin is a secondary protein structure consisting of two amino acid chains linked by two pairs of disulphide bridges. It is produced from preproinsulin (a prohormone) in the endoplasmic reticulum, where a portion is cleaved off and the remaining portion is folded with the aid of C-peptide to form proinsulin. The C-peptide fragment is then removed and the active insulin is transported via the Golgi apparatus to cytoplasmic granules for exocytosis into the plasma.

Once released, under the influence of many different stimuli, the insulin binds to its receptor on insulin-sensitive cells. The receptor is a tetramer consisting of two α and two β subunits. The insulin binds to the α subunit on the cell membrane surface while the β subunit spans the membrane and activates an intracellular second-messenger system via tyrosine kinase. Glucagon binding to its receptor activates a G-protein second-messenger system via adenylyl cyclase.

Receptor binding activates several cytoplasmic vesicles containing cell membrane transporter molecules. The vesicles fuse with the membrane, incorporating the transporter molecules. These molecules facilitate the movement of glucose into the cell. Once the insulin signal depletes these molecules are endocytosed back into the cell and recycled for re-use later.

Insulin also increases potassium entry into cells, and although the mechanism for this is not fully understood it is thought it may relate to increased Na^+/K^+-ATPase pump action. The effects of insulin on carbohydrate metabolism are to increase glucose entry into cells and increase glycogenesis. It is principally an anabolic hormone, increasing the storage of the metabolic breakdown products of carbohydrates, fats and proteins.

Smith T, Pinnock C, Lin T. *Fundamentals of Anaesthesia*, 3rd edn. Cambridge: Cambridge University Press, 2009; pp. 481.

MTF Question 54: Antidepressants as analgesics

Regarding the use of antidepressants for pain, which of the following statements are true?

a) The dose of amitriptyline to treat neuropathic pain is higher than the dose required to treat depression
b) The onset of analgesic action is slower than the onset of antidepressant action
c) Amitriptyline is licensed for use in neuropathic pain
d) Nortriptyline is less sedative than amitriptyline
e) Selective serotonin re-uptake inhibitors are more effective than the tricyclic antidepressants in treating pain

Answer: d

Short explanation

The dose of amitriptyline to treat pain is much lower than that required to treat depression and the onset of action is much faster. Amitriptyline is not licensed for use in neuropathic pain. Tricyclic antidepressants prevent the reuptake of monoamines, and these mixed reuptake drugs work better than more selective drugs.

Long explanation

The dose of amitriptyline to treat pain is much lower than that required to treat depression, and the onset of action is much faster; the antidepressant effect can take up to 2 weeks. Amitriptyline is not licensed for use in neuropathic pain, but it is a well-recognised indication with large trials to support its use.

Nortriptyline is less sedative than amitriptyline; however, the sedative effects of the tricyclic antidepressants can be helpful in treating sleep deprivation associated with chronic pain syndromes.

The tricyclic antidepressants prevent the reuptake of monoamines, including serotonin and noradrenaline, as both pathways are important in the pain propagation. The mixed reuptake drugs work better than more selective drugs.

Ryder S A, Stannard C F. Treatment of chronic pain: antidepressant, antiepileptic and antiarrhythmic drugs. *Contin Educ Anaesth Crit Care Pain* 2005; **5**: 18–20. Availble online at ceaccp.oxfordjournals.org/content/5/1/18 (accessed 15 March 2012).

MTF Question 55: Circle systems

Which of the following statements regarding circle systems are true?

a) Calcium hydroxide is found in soda lime and is re-formed during the reaction with carbon dioxide
b) Low-flow anaesthesia with a circle system is safe in patients who are intoxicated
c) A 500 g canister of soda lime can absorb > 120 L of carbon dioxide gas
d) Prolonged low-flow anaesthesia with sevoflurane produces proteinuria, glycosuria and enzymuria, which can be detrimental to patients with pre-existing biochemical evidence of renal dysfunction
e) During low-flow anaesthesia, carboxyhaemoglobin levels may approach 3–4%

Answer: e

Short explanation

The recirculation of gas in a circle system with soda lime results in re-formation of sodium hydroxide and recirculation of any exhaled gases, which may include toxic gases if the patient is intoxicated. 1 kg of soda lime can absorb > 120 L of CO_2. Any proteinuria, glycosuria or enzymuria that develops is of no clinical consequence, even in patients with renal disease.

Long explanation

Soda lime contains 94% calcium hydroxide, 5% sodium hydroxide, a small amount of potassium hydroxide, silica and a dying agent. During the reaction with CO_2 the sodium hydroxide is reformed as follows:

- $CO_2 + 2NaOH \rightarrow Na_2CO_3 + H_2O + Heat$
- $Na_2CO_3 + Ca(OH)_2 \rightarrow 2NaOH + CaCO_3$

An amount of 1 kg of soda lime can absorb > 120 L of carbon dioxide gas. Low-flow anaesthesia in a circle system allows for economy of volatile agents, heating and humidification of circulating gases, and it reduces environmental pollution. Expiration and recirculation of unwanted gases such as alcohol, acetone or carbon monoxide contraindicates the use of low-flow anaesthesia in patients who are intoxicated with alcohol, poisoned by carbon monoxide or suffering decompensated diabetic states.

In patients without poisoning, carbon monoxide, a byproduct of protein metabolism, can accumulate in a low-flow circle system, but levels are usually ≤ 4%. Prolonged low-flow anaesthesia with sevoflurane produces compound A, which causes acute tubular necrosis in rats at concentrations in excess of 250 ppm, a dose nearly 200 times that seen in clinical practice. Any proteinuria, glycosuria or enzymuria which does develop has not been shown to be associated with any clinical manifestations, even in patients with pre-existing renal disease.

Al-Shaikh B, Stacey S. *Essentials of Anaesthetic Equipment*, 2nd edn. Edinburgh: Churchill Livingstone, 2002; pp. 74–9.
Nunn G. Low-flow anaesthesia. *Contin Educ Anaesth Crit Care Pain* 2008; **8**: 1–4. Available online at ceaccp.oxfordjournals.org/content/8/1/1 (accessed 15 March 2012).

MTF Question 56: Cerebral vascular anatomy

Regarding the anatomy of the circle of Willis:

a) One-third of the blood supply is from internal carotid arteries
b) The anterior cerebral artery supplies the superior and medial parts of the cerebral hemispheres

c) The middle communicating artery joins the internal carotid artery and posterior cerebral artery
d) The middle cerebral artery supplies the lateral aspect of the cerebral hemispheres
e) The superior cerebellar artery is a branch of the posterior inferior cerebellar artery

Answer: b,d

Short explanation
The circle of Willis is a vital arterial structure that joins the two internal carotid arteries (two-thirds of the supply) with the two vertebral arteries to supply the contents of the cranium. The superior cerebellar artery is a branch of the basilar artery. There is no middle communicating artery.

Long explanation
The circle of Willis is a union of the two internal carotid arteries and the two vertebral arteries. Anteriorly, the internal carotid arteries give rise to the anterior and middle cerebral arteries. The anterior cerebral arteries are joined together by a single anterior communicating artery to create a circular structure. Posteriorly, the vertebral arteries travel into the cranium via the vertebral artery foramen and unite to form the single basilar artery that traverses anteriorly. Another important single artery that is created by the merger of the two vertebral arteries is the anterior spinal artery.

The basilar artery gives rise to a number of important paired branches. Posterior to anterior, these are: posterior inferior cerebellar artery, anterior inferior cerebellar artery, superior cerebellar artery. The basilar artery gives rise to the posterior cerebral arteries, which join the anterior part of the circle of Willis via the posterior communicating arteries.

The anterior cerebral artery supplies the superior and medial parts of the cerebral hemispheres. The middle cerebral artery supplies the lateral aspects, while the posterior cerebral artery supplies the occipital lobe and medial side of the temporal lobe. One of the evolutionary advantages of this type of vascular network is that with temporary occlusion to one of the major branches of the circle then there may be distal collateral flow via the communicating arteries.

The most vulnerable arteries for developing aneurysms, in descending order of vulnerability, are: anterior communicating artery, posterior communicating artery, middle cerebral artery, basilar tip, internal carotid artery.

Arthur P. Cerebral circulation. Encyclopedia.com. Available online at www.encyclopedia.com/doc/1G2-3435200087.html (accessed 15 March 2012).
Circle of Willis. WebAnatomy.net. Available online at webanatomy.net/anatomy/circle_of_willis.jpg (accessed 15 March 2012).

MTF Question 57: Inflammatory mediators

Which of the following statements regarding inflammatory mediators are correct?

a) Leukotrienes cause vasodilation
b) The kinin system mediates increased capillary permeability
c) Tumour necrosis factor is a cytokine produced mainly by granulocytes
d) Histamine is produced by basophils
e) Chemokines, such as interleukin 8, are involved in chemotaxis

Answers: b,d,e

Short explanation
Leukotrienes stimulate granulocyte migration to the site of injury. Tumour necrosis factor (TNF) is an inflammatory cytokine produced primarily by macrophages. These

are derived from mature monocytes, which are not granulocytes (basophils, neutrophils, eosinophils). Chemokines are a family of cytokines involved in chemotaxis.

Long explanation

The clinical signs of inflammation are heat, redness, swelling, pain and reduced function. The presence of these signs depends on three fundamental events: vasodilation, exudation and migration of leucocytes. Vasodilation results in an increase in blood supply to the area of injury, causing heat and redness. Increased capillary permeability is associated with the movement of molecules and plasma across the vascular endothelium. This results in oedema and stasis within the vasculature. Migration of leucocytes to the affected area is via chemotaxis. In addition to their role in phagocytosis, leucocytes release inflammatory mediators that maintain and develop the inflammatory response. These events are achieved by the actions of preformed plasma inflammatory mediators and mediators released from inflammatory cells.

Plasma-derived mediators. Bradykinin, produced by the kinin system, results in vasodilation and increased capillary permeability. Complement mediators, such as C3a and C5a, stimulate mast cell degranulation and the subsequent vasodilation and increased permeability observed with histamine. In addition, complement activates neutrophils and stimulates phagocyte migration. The coagulation cascade and fibrinolytic system are also involved in the inflammatory response. Coagulation forms a protective clot over the injured area. Fibrinolysis helps regulate the coagulation process as well as the activation of neutrophils and macrophages by fibrin degradation products.

Cell-derived mediators. Histamine is produced by basophils and mast cells. Release is associated with vasodilation and increased capillary permeability. Leukotrienes, also produced by basophils and mast cells, are involved in chemotaxis of granulocytes. Cytokines are a large family of signalling molecules used in cellular communication. Some cytokines play a role in the inflammatory response. Tumour necrosis factor (TNF) is produced by many cell types but primarily by macrophages. It activates endothelial cells and enhances phagocytosis. Chemokines (chemotactic cytokines) are a family of small cystein-rich cytokines that are involved in chemotaxis of inflammatory cells. Nitric oxide, produced by endothelial cells and macrophages, is a powerful vasodilator and smooth-muscle relaxant.

Smith T, Pinnock C, Lin T. *Fundamentals of Anaesthesia*, 3rd edn. Cambridge: Cambridge University Press, 2009; pp. 247–51.

Power I, Kam P. *Principles of Physiology for the Anaesthetist.* London: Arnold, 2001; pp. 272–4.

MTF Question 58: Olfactory receptors

Regarding olfactory receptors:

a) Olfactory receptors project through the cribiform plate in the sphenoid bone
b) Adjacent basal cells produce mucus
c) Chemoreceptors are directly triggered by odiferous chemicals in the airflow
d) Sustenacular cells continually produce more olfactory receptors
e) Olfactory receptors have a half-life of one month

Answer: e

Short explanation

The cribiform plate is in the ethmoid bone. Basal cells produce new receptors, and sustenacular cells are supportive columnar epithelium. Odiferous chemicals need to be dissolved in mucus to trigger receptors.

Long explanation

There are approximately 100 million olfactory receptors in the nasal epithelium. They are found in the olfactory epithelium on the roof of the nasal cavity, including the superior and upper middle conchae. There are three main cell types present. The olfactory receptors are specialised bipolar neurones with a long dendrite projecting to the surface, where multiple tiny cilia extend outwards embedded in mucus. They detect odiferous chemicals that have dissolved in the mucus and trigger these chemo-receptors. Impulses then follow the neurone through the cribiform plate of the ethmoid bone in the roof of the nasal cavity to the olfactory bulb. From here projections extend to cortical and limbic regions of the brain for processing. The primary olfactory area in the temporal lobe processes the impulse through important connections to the hypothalamus, thalamus and frontal cortex.

Basal cells are found adjacent and deep to the olfactory cells. They are unique in that they are replacing mature neurones, as they continually replace the olfactory neurones, which have a half-life of one month.

Columnar epithelium found between the receptors makes up the mucus epithelial lining and is known as the sustenacular or supporting cells. Olfactory (Bowman's) glands can be found in the connective tissue beneath the olfactory epithelium. They produce the mucus in which the chemicals dissolve to trigger the olfactory chemoreceptors.

The olfactory receptors are the first-order neurones of cranial nerve I; however, innervation of the olfactory epithelial cells from cranial nerve VII (facial nerve) explains the tears and sniffing evoked by some smells.

Tortora GJ, Grabowski SR. *Principles of Anatomy and Physiology*, 8th edn. New York, NY: HarperCollins, 1996; pp. 454–5.

MTF Question 59: Noradrenaline

The following physiological changes may be seen when commencing a noradrenaline infusion at 12 µg/minute:

a) Increased insulin secretion
b) Coronary vasodilation
c) Even with no change in perfusion pressure, renal blood flow will increase
d) Miosis
e) Pregnant uterine muscle relaxation

Answer: b

Short explanation

Noradrenaline decreases insulin secretion and renal blood flow, dilates the pupils and causes the pregnant uterus to contract.

Long explanation

Many anaesthetists use noradrenaline for sick patients and have a good idea of its major physiological effects. Examiners love the subtle differences that show that you have a mastery of the drugs you use.

Noradrenaline decreases insulin secretion and may produce hyperglycaemia. Noradrenaline vasodilates the coronary arteries. However, as myocardial work may increase, the balance of myocardial oxygen consumption and delivery may lead to ischaemia on noradrenaline. If pupillary changes occur in response to noradrenaline, mydriasis rather than miosis would be observed. The pregnant uterus will contract in response to a noradrenaline infusion. If the perfusion pressure of the kidneys is held constant, the effect of noradrenaline will be to decrease renal blood flow. It does not, however, have much effect on glomerular filtration rate.

Sasada M, Smith S. *Drugs in Anaesthesia and Intensive Care Part II*, 3rd edn. Oxford: Oxford Medical Publications, 2006; pp. 280–1.

MTF Question 60: Dietary lipids

The components of dietary lipids have different functions. Which of the following are true regarding the components of dietary lipid?

a) Fatty acids are the body's main form of stored energy
b) Fatty acid chains are stored in triglycerides
c) Triglycerides are transported free in the plasma
d) Lipoproteins have specific roles for different tissue targets
e) Phospholipids form structural components of cell membranes

Answer: a,b,d,e

Short explanation
Fatty acids are the individual components of triglycerides. Triglycerides form the central core of chylomicrons, which transport them round the body as lipoproteins. There are several types of lipoproteins, differing in structure. They target specific tissues.

Long explanation
Dietary lipids consist mainly of triglycerides. Triglycerides are fatty acids that are either saturated or unsaturated carbon chains of varied length with a carboxyl group on the end. Esterification, and the addition of glycerol catalysed by acetyl coenzyme A (acetyl-CoA) to these chains forms triglyceride. Like many components of dietary lipids they have important structural roles as well as being the main source of stored energy.

Triglycerides are broken down into their components to allow them to enter the intestinal epithelial cells. Once inside the cell they reform into triglycerides and combine with cholesterol, glucose and hydrophilic proteins to form the transport molecules, a chylomicron. Triglycerides are not transported freely in the plasma.

Of those lipids that are transported in the plasma 95% are combined with protein to form lipoproteins. The contents and density of these proteins determine their functions, but they each have specific roles for different tissues. For example, they are responsible for the transport of cholesterol to and from certain tissues in the body.

Phospholipids and glycolipids have important structural roles, contributing to the formation of the lipid bi-layer of cell membranes and tissues. The cholesterol component of dietary lipids has an essential role in the formation of steroid hormones and tissue membranes.

Smith T, Pinnock C, Lin T. *Fundamentals of Anaesthesia*, 3rd edn. Cambridge: Cambridge University Press, 2009; p. 461.

SBA Question 61: Critical temperature

Consider a hypothetical situation in which the following gases or vapours are stored separately in cylinders in a hot operating theatre (the thermometer reads 35 °C). Which one of the following would NOT contain gas alone, irrespective of the pressure within the cylinder?

a) Oxygen
b) Nitrogen
c) Nitrous oxide

d) Carbon dioxide
e) Air

Answer: c

Short explanation
Critical temperature (or pseudocritical temperature for a mixture of gases) is the temperature above which a vapour cannot be liquefied irrespective of how much pressure is applied. The critical temperatures of O_2, N_2, N_2O, CO_2 and air are $-118\,°C$, $-147\,°C$, $36.5\,°C$, $31\,°C$ and $-140.5\,°C$, respectively.

Long explanation
The critical temperature of a substance is the temperature above which a vapour cannot be liquefied irrespective of the amount of pressure that is applied. Interestingly enough, though, if you apply sufficiently high pressures you can form a solid. Remember that a vapour is defined as matter in gaseous form formed from a liquid but below its critical temperature. Similarly, a gas is matter formed by a liquid that is above its critical temperature.

The critical temperatures of the more common gases in anaesthesia are shown in the table. The critical temperatures of the volatile anaesthetic agents are of little relevance in everyday anaesthetic practice. These should not be confused with the boiling points, which are of relevance, particularly that of desflurane.

Gas	Critical temperature
Oxygen	$-118\,°C$
Nitrogen	$-147\,°C$
Nitrous oxide	$36.5\,°C$
Carbon dioxide	$31\,°C$
Air	$-140.5\,°C$

SBA Question 62: Materno-fetal drug distribution

You are asked to provide anaesthesia for a pregnant woman undergoing emergency appendicectomy. Of the following drugs administered to the woman, which is the least likely to accumulate in the fetus?

a) Bupivacaine
b) Pethidine
c) Thiopental
d) Diamorphine
e) Diazepam

Answer: a

Short explanation
Pethidine, diamorphine and diazepam are all metabolised to less lipid-soluble molecules which cannot cross back into the mother. Thiopental can accumulate because of rapid transfer and differential levels of protein binding. Bupivacaine can become ionised and trapped in the fetus, but only in significant acidosis.

Long explanation
The placenta forms a barrier to the transfer of drugs between the mother and the fetus but it is not particularly discriminating and most drugs will cross it to a certain degree. Factors which increase the rate of transfer include increasing lipid-solubility,

decreasing maternal protein binding, decreasing molecular weight, increased materno-fetal concentration gradient and placental blood flow.

Feto-maternal (F/M) concentration ratios describe the relative distribution of the drug across the placenta. Certain drugs may accumulate in the fetal tissue (i.e. have F/M ratios > 1) for several reasons. Highly lipid-soluble drugs such as thiopental cross the placenta easily, and can accumulate as the pH is lower in the fetus, causing differential rates of protein binding. Pethidine and diamorphine are both metabolised in the fetus to less lipid-soluble products (norpethidine and morphine, respectively) which remain on the fetal side of the placenta. The elimination half-lives of these drugs are also longer in the fetus because of immature hepatic metabolism, further prolonging their presence in the fetus. Diazepam is also metabolised to less lipid-soluble products, and can have an F/M ratio of 2 an hour after maternal administration.

Local anaesthetic agents are weak bases which are largely un-ionised at physiological pH, and hence cross the placenta readily. Bupivacaine has a higher degree of protein binding than other local anaesthetics (e.g. lidocaine), meaning that its rate of transfer is relatively low. If the fetus is markedly acidotic, increased ionisation in the fetus can cause 'ion trapping' and drug accumulation within the fetus. However, this is not clinically significant at normal pH values because the pKa of the drug (8.1) is well above the physiologically observed range.

Smith T, Pinnock C, Lin T. *Fundamentals of Anaesthesia*, 3rd edn. Cambridge: Cambridge University Press, 2009.

SBA Question 63: Principles of ventilators

A patient on the intensive care unit is being ventilated in a volume-controlled mode with an FiO_2 of 0.6. Arterial blood gas analysis reveals a PaO_2 of 7.5 kPa and a $PaCO_2$ of 4.7 kPa. Which ONE of the following is the best intervention aimed at increasing the PaO_2?

a) Increase the FiO_2
b) Increase the tidal volume
c) Increase the frequency
d) Increase the inspiratory time
e) Increase the expiratory time

Answer: d

Short explanation

The best intervention is one that increases the mean airway pressure (therefore addressing the cause of the hypoxia) without increasing the peak airway pressure or reducing the $PaCO_2$. This is best achieved by increasing the inspiration-to-expiration ratio and therefore increasing the inspiratory time.

Long explanation

Increasing the PaO_2 of a hypoxic patient is a common requirement for anaesthetists working in both theatre and the intensive care unit. The underlying principle here is that the PaO_2 is directly related to the mean airway pressure. Any intervention that increases the mean airway pressure will increase the PaO_2 by recruiting more alveoli. Increasing the expiratory time will result in proportionally more of the respiratory cycle being spent with low airway pressures – this will not be of benefit and may worsen the PaO_2. Increasing the tidal volume in volume-controlled ventilation will increase the peak airway pressure with only slight increases in the mean airway pressure. Increasing the frequency will again increase the mean airway pressure slightly, but will also increase the minute ventilation, which in this case will lower the $PaCO_2$ below its normal range. Increasing the FiO_2 increases the PaO_2 but does not address the reason behind the hypoxia.

Increasing the inspiratory time will increase the mean airway pressure and increase the PaO_2 by recruiting alveoli, thereby addressing the cause of the hypoxia. This is therefore the best intervention that can be performed in this situation, given the information presented.

SBA Question 64: Acute myocardial infarction

Regarding the management of acute myocardial infarction presenting with ischaemic symptoms and persistent ST elevation, which ONE of the following would be an absolute contraindication to fibrinolytic therapy?

a) Previous fibrinolysis 5 months ago
b) Resuscitated cardiac arrest within the last hour
c) Diabetic retinopathy
d) Ischaemic stroke 2 months ago
e) Pregnant at 36 weeks gestation

Answer: d

Short explanation
Previous fibrinolysis is not a contraindication as long as streptokinase is not used twice. Simple resuscitation and diabetic retinopathy are not contraindications, and pregnancy is only a relative contraindication.

Long explanation
After initial diagnosis and management with oxygen, analgesia and aspirin, coronary revascularisation is a priority in patients with ischaemic symptoms and persistent ST elevation (STEMI). Percutaneous coronary intervention is preferable, as it is more efficacious, but it cannot always be carried out expeditiously. If this is likely to be the case then it is better to give early fibrinolytic therapy.

Absolute contraindications to fibrinolysis are previous haemorrhagic stroke or stroke of unknown origin, ischaemic stroke in the previous 6 months, central nervous system trauma or neoplasia, major trauma, surgery or head injury within the preceding 3 weeks, gastrointestinal bleed within the last month, known bleeding disorder, aortic dissection, and recent non-compressible punctures such as liver biopsy or lumbar puncture. Relative contraindications include transient ischaemic attacks in the last 6 months, oral anticoagulant therapy, pregnancy or within 1 week postpartum, refractory hypertension (defined as systolic BP > 180 mmHg and/or diastolic BP > 110 mmHg), advanced liver disease, infective endocarditis, active peptic ulcer disease and refractory resuscitation.

Previous fibrinolysis is not a contraindication unless the previous and current regimens were both with streptokinase. The increasing use of tissue plasminogen activator (tPA) has made this less of a problem in recent years. Diabetic retinopathy and successful simple resuscitation from cardiac arrest are not contraindications to fibrinolysis.

European Society of Cardiology Guidelines. Available online at www.escardio.org/guidelines-surveys/esc-guidelines/GuidelinesDocuments/guidelines-AMI-FT.pdf (accessed 15 March 2012).

SBA Question 65: Diffusion across a membrane

A new drug is being tested. Its onset of action depends on the rate of diffusion across the cell membrane. The following factors increase the rate of diffusion of a substance across a biological membrane, EXCEPT which one?

a) Decreased molecular weight
b) Increased concentration gradient
c) Decreased solubility of a gas
d) Increased lipid solubility
e) For a weakly acidic substance, a low environmental pH

Answer: c

Short explanation

Diffusion increases with concentration gradient, lipid solubility and decreasing molecular weight. Weak acids are un-ionised in acidic conditions and hence more lipid-soluble. An insoluble gas will rapidly equilibrate its partial pressures across a membrane and therefore undergo less diffusion than a soluble gas.

Long explanation

Factors which increase the rate of diffusion across a membrane include:

- increased membrane surface area
- increased membrane permeability to the substance
- decreased molecular size or weight of the diffusing substance
- increased concentration or partial pressure gradient
- increased lipid-solubility and decreased water-solubility of the diffusing substance
- decreased polarity or ionisation of the diffusing substance
- (for ionised substances) an electrochemical gradient favouring the direction of diffusion

A weakly acidic substance will tend to be un-ionised in a low-pH environment, and therefore its diffusion will be enhanced. Where a membrane separates a gas from a fluid, the partial pressure of the gas is equivalent to its concentration and influences the rate of diffusion. The more soluble the gas, the more slowly the partial pressure rises in the liquid compartment, maintaining a pressure gradient and enhancing its transfer.

Yentis S, Hirsch N, Smith G. *Anaesthesia and Intensive Care A–Z: an Encyclopaedia of Principles and Practice*, 4th edn. Edinburgh: Butterworth–Heinemann, 2009.

SBA Question 66: Hormones

A hormone is produced in the cytoplasm of an endocrine cell and is then stored in granules within the cytoplasm. On release from the cell it is carried in the bloodstream to a target cell, where it crosses the cell membrane and binds directly to the nucleus, increasing cell gene transcription. Which hormone is best described in these terms?

a) Adrenaline
b) Thyroxine
c) Aldosterone
d) Thyroid-stimulating hormone
e) Growth hormone

Answer: b

Short explanation

This process describes an amine hormone synthesised within cellular cytoplasm and stored within granules. A subgroup of amine hormones are the thyroid hormones, which cross the cell membrane and act directly at the cell nucleus.

Long explanation

Hormones are chemical substances that are produced by an endocrine cell, secreted into blood and carried to a specific target cell where they bind with specific receptors and alter cellular action. There are three main classes of hormone: peptides, amines and steroids.

Peptides are synthesised in the cell nucleus and are then stored in granules and released by exocytosis. Amines are synthesised in the cytoplasm and then stored in granules. Steroid hormones are synthesised from cholesterol and immediately released without storage.

Peptide hormones (e.g. growth hormone) act via second messengers to alter cellular functions.

Amine hormones are sub-classified into catecholamines (e.g. adrenaline), which act at cell membranes by second messengers, and thyroid hormones (e.g. thyroxine), which bind directly to nucleus receptors, stimulating transcription.

Steroid hormones are lipid-soluble. They enter the cytoplasm, bind with protein receptors in the cytoplasm and then enter the nucleus to stimulate transcription.

Power I, Kam P. *Principles of Physiology for the Anaesthetist.* London: Arnold, 2001; pp. 283–5.

SBA Question 67: Cardiac output measurement

A 52-year-old male with no comorbidities is undergoing a right hemicolectomy for bowel carcinoma. His pulse is 70 beats/min, his blood pressure is 90/55 mmHg. An oesophageal Doppler displays the following variables: cardiac output 4.2 L/min, stroke volume 43 mL, flow time corrected (FTc) 300, peak velocity (PV) 55 cm/second. Which ONE of the following would be the best intervention?

a) Start an infusion of dopexamine
b) Start an infusion of dobutamine
c) Give a 200 mL fluid challenge
d) Start an infusion of noradrenaline
e) Give a 500 mL fluid challenge

Answer: c

Short explanation

The case suggests a patient with a reduced cardiac output, stroke volume, FTc and PV. The most appropriate initial step would be a 200 mL fluid challenge with observation of the response. Only following an absence of a 10% improvement in these values should inotropic or vasodilatory support be considered.

Long explanation

Patients undergoing colorectal surgery are susceptible to large fluid shifts, which may result in occult hypovolaemia. The subsequent hypoperfusion of the gastrointestinal tract may result in reduced oxygen delivery, which puts patients at risk of gastro-intestinal morbidity and increased hospital stay. The use of a cardiac output monitor in this setting has been shown to assist in guiding intraoperative fluid prescription and avoiding these sequelae. The oesophageal Doppler is one such cardiac output monitor, and there is evidence to support its use in this setting.

Interpretation of the above values requires knowledge of the normal ranges and their physiological relationships. The normal ranges for a 52-year-old male with no comorbidities are:

- Cardiac output 5–8 L/min
- Stroke volume 55–100 mL

- PV 70–100 cm/second
- FTc 330–360 milliseconds

The flow time can be conceptualised as the time taken for the stroke volume to travel past the probe. The flow time will clearly vary according to the heart rate, and so, to compare it more appropriately to the other measured variables, the flow time is corrected to a heart rate of 60 beats per minute to give the flow time corrected (FTc). The FTc is inversely related to the systemic vascular resistance. PV is directly related to the left ventricular contractility and the number is age-dependent.

Putting all the data together suggests a man who may be underfilled despite an acceptable blood pressure and pulse. The most appropriate intervention would be to administer a fluid challenge of 200 mL and observe the change in the measured variables above. An increase in the stroke volume or stroke distance of > 10% would be seen as a positive response and the challenge should be repeated. Failure to respond to fluid should only then lead to consideration of inotropic agents and possibly vasodilators.

Wakeling HG, McFall MR, Jenkins CS, *et al*. Intraoperative oesophageal Doppler guided fluid management shortens postoperative hospital stay after major bowel surgery. *Br J Anaesth* 2005; **95**: 634–42.

Deltex Medical Group Guide for using Cardio Q in the OR (2010). Available online at www.deltexmedical.com/downloads/clinicaleducationguides/CQ_OR_QRG90 51_5309_3.pdf (accessed 15 March 2012).

SBA Question 68: Narrow-complex tachycardia

An adult patient in the recovery room develops a narrow-complex AV nodal re-entry tachycardia. The patient has an acceptable blood pressure and no signs of myocardial ischaemia or heart failure. Vagal manoeuvres followed by a rapid 6 mg bolus of intravenous adenosine have failed to change the rhythm. Which of the following would represent the best practice for immediate ongoing management?

a) Anaesthetise and perform DC cardioversion
b) Administer 12 mg of intravenous adenosine
c) Administer 300 mg of intravenous amiodarone
d) Administer 2.5 mg of intravenous verapamil
e) Administer 5 mg of intravenous metoprolol

Answer: b

Short explanation
The 2010 Resuscitation Council Guidelines state that in this scenario the next course of action would be to administer a 12 mg rapid bolus of adenosine, and if this failed to work to administer a second 12 mg dose of adenosine.

Long explanation
Narrow-complex tachycardias are usually sinus tachycardia, AV nodal re-entry, AV re-entry or atrial flutter with regular conduction. It is important to determine that the narrow-complex tachycardia is not a sinus rhythm, as drug therapy would then be likely to make the patient's condition worse.

The 2010 Resuscitation Council Guidelines state that the initial management of a patient with a narrow-complex AV nodal re-entry tachycardia is to perform vagal manoeuvres, and if that fails to administer a 6 mg dose of adenosine as a rapid bolus, ideally into a large central vein. If the rhythm remains unchanged, two further attempts with intravenous adenosine to convert the patient should be made, using the higher, 12 mg dose.

The vast majority of re-entry tachycardias will convert back into a sinus rhythm with vagal manoeuvres or adenosine. Failure to do so would usually indicate that the rhythm is an atrial tachycardia such as atrial flutter. If this is the case, rate control with a β-blocker would be the next course of action. Verapamil can be used in this scenario instead of adenosine, if adenosine is contraindicated.

Resuscitation Council Guidelines, 2010. Peri-arrest arrhythmias. Available online at www.resus.org.uk/pages/periarst.pdf (accessed 15 March 2012).

SBA Question 69: Visual pathway

An elderly man is admitted into the medical admission unit with a sudden deterioration in vision. Examination of the visual fields reveals loss of vision in only the right side of the visual field in both eyes (right homonymous hemianopia). Where in the visual pathway is the lesion?

a) Right optic nerve
b) Left optic nerve
c) Optic chiasm
d) Right optic radiation
e) Left optic radiation

Answer: e

Short explanation
The right-sided homonymous hemianopia is consistent with a lesion in the left optic radiation. Action potentials from the left (ipsilateral) temporal field and the right (contralateral) nasal field travel in the optic radiation to the left primary visual cortex, carrying information about the right visual field.

Long explanation
The visual pathway begins at the retina, where light reaches photoreceptors and initiates action potentials. Axons form the optic nerve at the blind spot on the optic disc, from where the nerve fibres travel to the optic chiasm. At the optic chiasm the axons in the optic nerve divide into fibres from the temporal half of the retina, which remain ipsilateral, and fibres from the nasal half of the retina, which decussate and continue in the visual path on the contralateral side. Thus lesions of the visual field at the optic chiasm classically result in a bi-temporal hemianopia (loss of vision in both eyes in the temporal portions of the visual field).

After the optic chiasm the nerve fibres travel in the optic tract to synapse at the lateral geniculate body. The visual pathway continues as the optic radiation, with action potentials from the ipsilateral temporal field and contralateral nasal field travelling to the primary visual cortex. Lesions at this point cause a homonymous hemianopia. A lesion in the left optic radiation causes blindness in the right visual field of both the right eye (contralateral nasal field) and left eye (ispilateral temporal field).

Smith T, Pinnock C, Lin T. *Fundamentals of Anaesthesia*, 3rd edn. Cambridge: Cambridge University Press, 2009; p. 405.

SBA Question 70: Temperature

You are discussing with a colleague anatomical sites used to measure core temperature in a patient under anaesthesia. Which of your colleague's following statements regarding temperature measurement is NOT correct?

a) The tympanic membrane is a useful site from which to sample temperature, as it closely correlates with hypothalamic temperature and has a rapid response time
b) Temperature sampled from the upper third of the oesophagus accurately reflects core body temperature
c) Bladder temperature measurement is more accurate at high urine flow rates than low urine flow rates
d) Rectal temperature is usually 0.5–1 °C higher than core body temperature
e) Core body temperature is measured accurately and continuously from the pulmonary artery

Answer: b

Short explanation
Oesophageal temperature is only accurate when sampled from the lower third of the oesophagus; sampling from the upper third may prove inaccurate.

Long explanation
Temperature may be sampled from the tympanic membrane, oesophagus, nasopharynx, bladder, rectum, skin and blood.

The tympanic membrane accurately reflects hypothalamic temperature and has a rapid response time, unlike the rectum, which is hotter than core temperature owing to bacterial fermentation and has a delayed response time owing to insulation by faeces. The oesophagus is accurate if the lower third is used. The upper third is influenced by the temperature of inspired gases. Bladder temperature is influenced by urinary flow rates, with high flow rates being needed for the measurement to accurately reflect true core temperature. Pulmonary artery catheters have integral thermistors that accurately and continuously measure temperature in the pulmonary artery.

The radiant intensity of a body is governed by the Stefan–Boltzmann law. This law describes how the total amount of radiation from a body is proportional to the fourth power of the body's absolute temperature. Therefore a kitchen oven that is twice room temperature (600 compared to 300 kelvin) radiates 16 times as much power per unit area. The constant of proportionality here is the Stefan–Boltzmann constant.

Yentis S, Hirsch N, Smith G. *Anaesthesia and Intensive Care A–Z: an Encyclopaedia of Principles and Practice*, 3rd edn. Edinburgh: Butterworth–Heinemann, 2004; pp. 503–4.

SBA Question 71: Endurance training

You have been training hard for over a year in preparation for an 'Ironman' triathlon race in Switzerland in the summer. You would expect all of the following changes to occur with this endurance training, EXCEPT which one?

a) Significant increase in the resting stroke volume as well as maximal exercise stroke volume
b) Increased resting oxygen uptake, from 0.3 L/min to 0.5 L/min
c) Increased maximum oxygen uptake, from 2.8 L/min to 5.2 L/min
d) Hypertrophy of the heart, which is similar to the effects of hypertension
e) Delayed exercise-related rise in lactate

Answer: b

Short explanation

Resting oxygen uptake does not change with training, although oxygen uptake is achieved by increasing the VO_2 max. VO_2 (oxygen uptake) is equal to the oxygen delivered minus the oxygen returned.

Long explanation

Training increases and maintains capacity to do physical exercise. As exercise intensity increases, so does fuel consumption and type of fuel used. The first few minutes of exercise utilise creatine phosphate and glycogen. Oxidation of glucose and free fatty acids enables effective aerobic exercise. During prolonged or strenuous exercise, anaerobic metabolism provides additional energy at the expense of producing lactate. Aerobic threshold is approximately equal to a lactate concentration of 2 mmol/L and can be tolerated for a reasonable period of time. When anaerobic threshold is reached at 4 mmol/L of lactate, this is the point at which performance rapidly declines.

The level at which maximum oxygen consumption occurs is VO_2 max, and it is effort-dependent. The rate of rise of lactate is slower in trained athletes. Endurance training increases the oxidative capacity of slow-twitch muscle units by increasing the number of mitochondria. This increase in mitochondria in combination with an increase in cardiac output increases the VO_2 max. The VO_2 max is limited by cardiovascular capacity, not by respiratory capacity, in healthy individuals.

Training alters the morphology of the heart by hypertrophy of the myocardium. Although this is morphologically similar to the changes that occur with chronic hypertension, the athletic heart does not demonstrate diastolic dysfunction. The resting stroke volume increases from approximately 70 mL in an untrained male to 140 mL in an athletic male. In order to maintain the same resting cardiac output, the athlete's resting pulse decreases from 80 to 40 beats/min. The maximal stroke volume achieved during exercise also increases with training from 100 mL to 190 mL in males. Trained athletes work out at a higher maximal stroke volume, which therefore enables the heart to work more efficiently at a lower pulse rate compared with untrained individuals.

Despopoulos A, Silbernagl S. *Color Atlas of Physiology*, 5th edn. New York, NY: Thieme, 2003; pp. 74–7.

Suleman A, Riaz K, Heffner KD. Exercise physiology. *Medscape Reference* 2008. Available online at emedicine.medscape.com/article/88484 (accessed 15 March 2012).

SBA Question 72: Capacitance

Whilst in theatre with an anaesthetised, intubated and ventilated patient, you notice interference on your ECG trace. What would be the most likely explanation for this interference?

a) The patient must be in contact with live electrical equipment
b) Direct current can pass from a theatre lamp
c) Electrons can flow directly across an air gap
d) The patient can behave like one plate of a capacitor
e) The patient is moving

Answer: d

Short explanation

The patient can indeed behave like one plate of a capacitor, with an electric lamp, for example, acting as the other plate. The ability of an alternating (but not direct) current to pass across an air gap because of capacitance explains why electrical interference may appear on your ECG trace. Hopefully, if your patients are intubated and ventilated, they do not move sufficiently to disrupt your ECG trace!

Long explanation

Capacitance is a measure of the ability of an object to store electric charge. Charge is a measure of the amount of electricity and is measured in coulombs (C). The coulomb is the quantity of electric charge which passes some point when a current of one ampere flows for a period of one second. The unit of capacitance is the farad, one farad being the capacity to store one coulomb of charge for an applied potential difference of one volt.

A capacitor consists of two plates (conductors) separated by an insulator (air), and it can be charged when a potential difference flows across it. A capacitor cannot conduct electrons directly across the gap between the plates and therefore a direct current will not be able to flow. If an alternating current is allowed to pass, it will continuously be being charged and discharged, so allowing a current to flow.

This ability of alternating current to pass across an air gap because of capacitance explains why you can see electrical interference on the ECG trace. This can occur if, for example, an operating theatre lamp is separated from a patient by an air gap: the patient and the lamp each forms a plate. As a small mains-frequency current passes from the lamp to the patient a 50 Hz voltage can appear on the ECG, and this may be sufficient to obscure the reading. As you well know, there are several other forms of interference that can occur to upset your ECG trace!

Davis PD, Kenny GNC. *Basic Physics and Measurement in Anaesthesia*, 5th edn. Oxford: Butterworth–Heinemann, 2003; p. 159.
Yentis S, Hirsch N, Smith G. *Anaesthesia and Intensive Care A–Z: an Encyclopaedia of Principles and Practice*, 4th edn. Edinburgh: Butterworth–Heinemann, 2009; p. 85.

SBA Question 73: Starling forces

A 80-year-old woman is treated for New York Heart Association (NYHA) class II heart failure. On a routine visit to her GP she is noted to have palpable pitting oedema to her mid calf. Which of the following best describes the mechanism by which this is occurring?

a) Increased proximal capillary hydrostatic pressure
b) Increased distal capillary hydrostatic pressure
c) Decreased proximal capillary hydrostatic pressure
d) Decreased distal capillary hydrostatic pressure
e) Increased interstitial hydrostatic pressure

Answer: b

Short explanation

Congestive cardiac failure causes a rise in venous pressure. This raises the distal capillary hydrostatic pressure, reducing reabsorption of fluid in the venous capillary (thus an increase in net filtration), leading to an excess of interstitial fluid and the development of oedema.

Long explanation

The movement of fluid in and out of capillaries is determined by the balance of hydrostatic pressures in the capillary and interstitium and the colloid osmotic pressures in the capillary and interstitium. A variety of pathological states alter the equilibrium and oedema results.

In a normal state the hydrostatic pressure from arterial end to venous end of the capillary falls from approximately 33 mmHg to 15 mmHg, and interstitial hydrostatic pressure is around 1 mmHg (in solid organs). The colloid osmotic pressure is around 25 mmHg in the capillary and zero in the interstitial fluid.

Thus at the arterial end of the capillary there is a net filtration because the capillary hydrostatic pressure forcing fluid out of the vessels exceeds the capillary colloid pressure and interstitial hydrostatic pressure, encouraging fluid reabsorption: $33 - (25 + 1) = +7$.

At the venous end of the capillary there is net reabsorption, because there is less capillary hydrostatic pressure: $15 - (25 + 1) = -11$.

In the pathological state of heart failure the capillary venous pressure is raised to above 15 mmHg, and thus reabsorption is reduced, net filtration increases, fluid accumulates and oedema occurs.

Smith T, Pinnock C, Lin T. *Fundamentals of Anaesthesia*, 3rd edn. Cambridge: Cambridge University Press, 2009; pp. 308–9.

SBA Question 74: Flow

Which of the following is the most accurate description of the flow in a Rotameter?

a) It demonstrates turbulent flow throughout
b) It demonstrates laminar flow throughout
c) It demonstrates variable pressure throughout
d) For any given flow rate setting, the Reynolds number increases towards the top of the Rotameter
e) Calibration depends on both density and viscosity

Answer: e

Short explanation

The Rotameter is a constant-pressure, variable-orifice flowmeter. There is a mixture of turbulent and laminar flow, so for calibration purposes both density and viscosity are important. Reynolds number may be under or over 2000, depending on whether flow is laminar or turbulent.

Long explanation

Flow is the amount of fluid, either liquid or gas, passing a point per unit time. There are two types of flow: laminar and turbulent.

Laminar flow is normally present in smooth tubes at low rates of flow and demonstrates smooth patterns with no eddies or turbulence. The flow is greatest in the centre, being almost double the mean flow, and at the edge of the tube the flow approaches zero. Laminar flow obeys the Hagen–Poiseuille equation stating that flow is proportional to the pressure difference and the fourth power of the radius and inversely proportional to the length of the tube and the viscosity.

Turbulent flow occurs in uneven-shaped tubes, around corners or when laminar flow velocity is too fast, exceeding the critical velocity. It flows in eddies and the resistance is higher than for the same laminar flow. Turbulent flow is proportional to the radius squared and the square root of the pressure gradient and is indirectly proportional to the length of the tube and density of the fluid.

Reynolds number is a dimensionless number which allows us to predict if a flow is likely to be laminar or turbulent. If it is less than 2000 flow is likely to be laminar, and if it is greater than 2000 it is likely to be turbulent.

The Rotameter is an example of a constant-pressure variable-orifice flowmeter, and it is used on anaesthetic machines to allow us to measure the flow of gases. A bobbin is supported in a tapered tube by gas flow and, as the flow increases, the bobbin rises in the tube. There is a variable orifice around the bobbin that depends on the gas flow. The pressure across the bobbin remains constant. There is a mixture of laminar and turbulent flow, so calibration depends on both the density and viscosity of the gas.

At low flow rates, the bobbin sits low down in the rotameter and the flow around the sides is laminar. As the flow rate rises, so does the bobbin. Flow passing around the bobbin travels through an orifice rather than a tube and becomes turbulent.

Davis PD, Kenny GNC. *Basic Physics and Measurement in Anaesthesia*, 5th edn. Oxford: Butterworth–Heinemann, 2003; pp. 11–12, 26–7.

Yentis S, Hirsch N, Smith G. *Anaesthesia and Intensive Care A–Z: an Encyclopaedia of Principles and Practice*, 4th edn. Edinburgh: Butterworth–Heinemann, 2009; pp. 210–11.

SBA Question 75: Abnormal Valsalva responses

An abnormal Valsalva response may be detected when assessing patients with a number of pathological conditions such as diabetic peripheral neuropathy. Which of the following statements about abnormal Valsalva responses is INCORRECT?

a) Autonomic dysfunction causes the blood pressure to fall and remain low until phase III
b) A square-wave response may be seen in hypovolaemic patients
c) No change in heart rate is observed in patients with autonomic dysfunction
d) The blood pressure rises but does not fall in patients with cardiac tamponade
e) Abnormal Valsalva can be demonstrated after sympathectomy

Answer: b

Short explanation

Hypovolaemic patients may demonstrate an exaggerated drop in blood pressure. A 'square wave' response is seen in conditions with elevated central venous pressure such as cardiac failure, constrictive pericarditis and cardiac tamponade.

Long explanation

Antonio Maria Valsalva (1666–1723) was an Italian anatomist who first described this manoeuvre for clearing blocked eustachian tubes. Abnormal responses to Valsalva can be demonstrated in a number of conditions. Assessment of Valsalva response is a useful and easy bedside test of autonomic function.

A number of conditions can cause autonomic neuropathy. Central causes of autonomic neuropathy include progressive autonomic failure (Shy–Drager syndrome), stroke and drugs. The most common cause of peripheral autonomic neuropathy is diabetes mellitus. Other causes include Guillian–Barré syndrome, porphyria and amyloidosis.

With autonomic neuropathy, there is a persisting fall in blood pressure secondary to the sustained high intrathoracic pressure. The baroreceptor reflexes fail to mediate a tachycardic response. When the intrathoracic pressure is released, there is no observed overshoot of blood pressure. The 'square wave' response is seen in conditions with elevated central venous pressure such as cardiac failure, constrictive pericarditis and cardiac tamponade. The blood pressure rises and remains elevated throughout phase II and then returns to normal. Provided that the vagus nerves remain intact to mediate reflex activity, a normal Valsalva response can be demonstrated after sympathectomy.

Smith T, Pinnock C, Lin T. *Fundamentals of Anaesthesia*, 3rd edn. Cambridge: Cambridge University Press, 2009; pp. 317–18.

A page on normal Valsalva manoeuvre is available online at www.cvphysiology.com/ Hemodynamics/H014.htm (accessed 15 March 2012).

SBA Question 76: Compensated respiratory acidosis

A patient with chronic obstructive pulmonary disease (COPD) presents for assessment for long-term oxygen therapy (LTOT) and is found to have a compensated respiratory acidosis. Which of the following sets of arterial blood gases best demonstrates compensated respiratory acidosis?

a) pH = 7.30, PCO_2 = 7.2 kPa, PO_2 = 9.5 kPa, HCO_3^- = 25 mmol/L
b) pH = 7.36, PCO_2 = 8.5 kPa, PO_2 = 7.5 kPa, HCO_3^- = 43 mmol/L
c) pH = 7.24, PCO_2 = 10.1 kPa, PO_2 = 7.0 kPa, HCO_3^- = 27 mmol/L
d) pH = 7.24, PCO_2 = 3.5 kPa, PO_2 = 8.5 kPa, HCO_3^- = 18 mmol/L
e) pH = 7.20, PCO_2 = 6.2 kPa, PO_2 = 9.0 kPa, HCO_3^- = 15 mmol/L

Answer: b

Short explanation

The first option shows acute uncompensated respiratory acidosis. The third is an example of acute on chronically compensated respiratory acidosis that is typical of an exacerbation of COPD. The fourth option demonstrates metabolic acidosis, and the last shows mixed respiratory and metabolic acidosis.

Long explanation

Respiratory acidosis is caused by an increase in $PaCO_2$ because the lungs are unable to remove the excess CO_2 from the body. There are many causes of hypercapnia (defined as $PaCO_2 > 6$ kPa), but a common cause is hypoventilation.

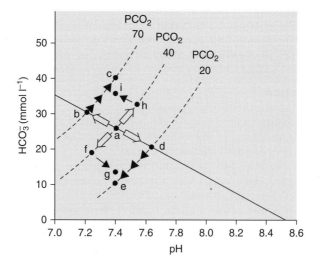

The increase in $PaCO_2$ causes a decrease in the ratio of HCO_3^-/PCO_2 (prior to effective renal compensation), thereby decreasing pH. Full renal compensation does not achieve a completely normal plasma pH of 7.4, but usually has a more typical value of 7.36.

Another useful value on arterial blood gas analysis is the 'base excess', which increases with renal compensation. The definition of base excess, or deficit, is the amount of acid or base (mmol) that is required to correct one litre of blood to a normal pH that is standardised to a $PaCO_2$ of 5.3 kPa (40 mmHg) and body temperature.

In acute hypercapnia the bicarbonate concentration should increase by approximately 0.7 mmol/L per 1 kPa rise in $PaCO_2$ (or 1 mmol/L per 10 mmHg). For chronic compensation, it is approximately four times the expected increase, at 2.6 mmol/L per 1 kPa rise in $PaCO_2$ (4 mmol/L per 10 mmHg). In COPD, patients who are 'CO_2 retainers' have a chronically compensated respiratory acidosis. During an exacerbation of COPD, which may or may not be infective, there will often be an acute-on-chronic respiratory acidosis. With an acute exacerbation, the bicarbonate level, pH and base excess will be lower compared with the patient's normal baseline blood gas. This is illustrated by the third option, which can be compared with the second as the patient's baseline blood gas.

A good example of mixed respiratory and metabolic acidosis is a patient who presents with an 'acute abdomen'. The cause may be ischaemic small bowel, so a lactic acidosis would be observed. Normally, hyperventilating and the subsequent hypo-capnia would compensate for this. However, if the patient's diaphragm becomes splinted secondary to abdominal distension, then the patient is unable to ventilate adequately to compensate, causing hypercapnia particularly as the patient tires.

Grogono AW. Interactive acid–base diagram: PCO_2 vs. SBE. Available online at www.acid-base.com/diagram.php (accessed 15 March 2012).

Kaufman DA. Interpretation of arterial blood gases (ABGs). American Thoracic Society. Available online at www.thoracic.org/clinical/critical-care/clinical-education/abgs.php (accessed 15 March 2012).

Smith T, Pinnock C, Lin T. *Fundamentals of Anaesthesia*, 3rd edn. Cambridge: Cambridge University Press, 2009; pp. 354–5.

SBA Question 77: Antiemetics and PONV risk

Consider anaesthetising 100 identical patients who were all 50-year-old non-smokers with a strong previous history of postoperative nausea and vomiting (PONV) scheduled for a total abdominal hysterectomy. You are likely to use an opioid for intraoperative and postoperative analgesia. How many of the 100 would be prevented from suffering PONV by the intraoperative administration of 4 mg intravenous ondansetron?

a) 5
b) 10
c) 20
d) 50
e) 80

Answer: c

Short explanation
With four risk factors, 78 out of the 100 patients will be at risk of PONV. Ondansetron will prevent PONV in 26% of the at-risk group. This would be 20 patients.

Long explanation
It is important to know the risk factors for PONV when considering administering or prescribing antiemetics. Risk factors for PONV were analysed and simplified in a seminal 1999 paper by Apfel *et al.*, which proposed a simple score containing just four factors. This scoring system has been further validated in a number of papers since publication.

The factors predicting risk of PONV were female gender, non-smoking, the use of postoperative opioids, and previous history of PONV or motion sickness. Depending on the presence of none, one, two, three or all four risk factors, the predicted probability of PONV would be 10%, 21%, 39%, 61% or 78%, respectively. There was an association between type of operation and PONV but this was thought to be due to the incidence of high-risk patients in the operative group rather than any causal relationship. For example, gynaecological surgery patients are female. Duration of surgery over 1 hour was shown to confer an increased risk but is a less useful predictor as it can often only be assessed retrospectively.

The 2004 paper by Apfel *et al.* demonstrated that a dose of ondansetron produces a relative risk reduction of 26%. So, in our scenario, 78% are at risk of PONV. Of the at-risk group, 26% are relieved by ondansetron perioperatively, so the number protected from PONV would be 20.

Apfel C, Laara E, Koivuranta M, Greim C, Roewer N. A simplified risk score for predicting postoperative nausea and vomiting. *Anesthesiology* 1999; **91**: 693–700.

Apfel CC, Korttila K, Abdalla M, *et al.*; IMPACT Investigators. A factorial trial of six interventions for the prevention of postoperative nausea and vomiting. *N Engl J Med* 2004; **350**: 2441–51.

SBA Question 78: Humoral control of haemorrhage

Which of the following statements regarding humoral mechanisms involved in controlling haemorrhage is INCORRECT?

a) Circulating catecholamines increase
b) Atrial natriuretic peptide (ANP) levels increase
c) Vasopressin release is mediated via the Gauer–Henry reflex
d) Stimulation of the adrenal cortex promotes release of aldosterone
e) Circulating levels of enkephalins increase

Answer: b

Short explanation

Release of atrial natriuretic peptide (ANP) is stimulated by atrial myocytes in response to atrial distension. It causes natriuresis, inhibition of antidiuretic hormone (ADH, vasopressin) secretion and also lowers blood pressure. During haemorrhage, levels of ANP will therefore decrease.

Long explanation

There are six compensatory mechanisms that are classically described for circulatory control of haemorrhage: baroreceptor reflexes, chemoreceptor reflexes, cerebral ischaemic response, reabsorption of tissue fluid into the plasma compartment, release of endogenous catecholamines, renal conservation of salt and water.

Activation of the sympathetic nervous system via the baroreceptor and chemoreceptor reflexes stimulates the adrenal medulla to increase catecholamines. The primary role of adrenaline is to augment cardiac contractility (via β_1) in order to maintain adequate cardiac output during haemorrhage. At low concentrations, adrenaline will cause skeletal vasodilation via β-adrenergic fibres, but at high concentration α-adrenergic-mediated vasoconstriction predominates. Noradrenaline is a potent vasoconstrictor whose release is mediated via sympathetic nerve endings as opposed to stimulation of the adrenal medulla.

Vasoconstriction is essential to maintain mean arterial blood pressure (MAP). Enkephalins are endogenous opioids that are contained in secretory granules with catecholamines. Levels of enkephalins are increased when the adrenal medulla is stimulated. Reduced perfusion of the juxtaglomerular apparatus stimulates renin release. This causes a cascade of events whereby renin converts plasma angiotensinogen to angiotensin I, which then becomes the potent vasoconstrictor angiotensin II. Angiotensin II stimulates the adrenal cortex to secrete aldosterone, which causes retention of sodium and attempts to maintain intravascular volume. Atrial stretch receptors detect a decrease in intravascular volume because atrial filling is reduced.

The stretch receptors transmit signals to stop secretion of atrial natriuretic peptide (ANP) and instead stimulate the release of antidiuretic hormone (ADH, vasopressin) from the posterior pituitary lobe, via the Gauer–Henry reflex. ADH is a potent vasoconstrictor in its own right, acting on V_1 receptors, and causes fluid retention via V_2 receptors.

Despopoulos A, Silbernagl S. *Color Atlas of Physiology*, 5th edn. New York, NY: Thieme, 2003; pp. 218–19.

Smith T, Pinnock C, Lin T. *Fundamentals of Anaesthesia*, 3rd edn. Cambridge: Cambridge University Press, 2009; pp. 311–12, 316–17.

SBA Question 79: Capnography

Capnography is part of the AAGBI minimal monitoring requirements for general anaesthesia. Regarding capnography, which of following is the LEAST correct?

a) Capnography is based on the principle that gases with two or more different atoms in the molecule will absorb infrared radiation
b) The particular frequency of infrared radiation is selected by first passing it through a crystal window
c) A reference cell increases accuracy of the system
d) The use of infrared radiation with a wavelength of 4.28 μm for the analysis of carbon dioxide should reduce interference from the presence of nitrous oxide
e) In the sidestream capnograph, a sample is drawn at about 150 mL/min

Answer: b

Short explanation
The particular frequency of infrared radiation is selected by first passing it through a filter. The sample chamber does have windows made from a material which is transparent to infrared radiation, such as a sapphire; glass absorbs infrared radiation.

Long explanation
Capnography is a vital part of patient monitoring under anaesthesia. It provides a continuous recording of carbon dioxide concentration and can be an early warning of problems under anaesthesia. Gases with two or more different atoms in the molecule can absorb infrared radiation, and by measuring the fraction of infrared absorbed by a gas, the concentration can be determined. Gases absorb infrared at particular wavelengths, and the proportion absorbed depends on the wavelength. Knowing the wavelengths for each gas in a mixture can help to prevent interference from unwanted gases; for example, using infrared with a wavelength of 4.28 μm for carbon dioxide reduces interference from nitrous oxide.

The infrared source is usually a hot wire, and the desired frequency is obtained by passing the radiation through a specific filter. The sample chamber has windows made of sapphire, as glass will absorb the radiation. Once it has passed through the sample chamber it is focused on a photodetector. The greater the absorption of the radiation, the less radiation reaches the photodetector. This can then be converted to an electronic output. Some instruments use a second beam of radiation which is passed through a reference chamber containing carbon-dioxide-free air, acting to avoid variations from the output source.

There are two types of capnograph: the sidestream and mainstream. In the sidestream, a sample is drawn at about 150 mL/min from a connector at the patient's airway and carried to the analyser. A trap prevents build-up of moisture, and gases are returned to the breathing system via an exhaust. This transit time to the analyser will delay the reading slightly but the tubing is designed to reduce this to a minimum, resulting in a delay of typically less than 1 second. The mainstream analyser incorporates a channel with sapphire windows that sits over the airway and passes a beam directly through the gases in the airway. This avoids transit time but is bulkier.

An accurate capnograph will have a rapid response time. This has two components: the transit time and the rise time. The rise time represents the time taken for the analyser to respond to the signal. This depends on the size of the sample chamber and the gas flow. Infrared analysers can also be used to measure other gases, such as nitrous oxide and other anaesthetic agents.

Davis PD, Kenny GNC. *Basic Physics and Measurement in Anaesthesia*, 5th edn. Oxford: Butterworth–Heinemann, 2003; pp. 214–17.
Yentis S, Hirsch N, Smith G. *Anaesthesia and Intensive Care A–Z: an Encyclopaedia of Principles and Practice*, 4th edn. Edinburgh: Butterworth–Heinemann, 2009; p. 85.

SBA Question 80: Local anaesthetic plasma levels

When a standard dose of lidocaine without vasoconstrictor is injected into various different sites around the body, care is taken to avoid intravascular injection and peak plasma levels of lidocaine are measured after injection. Which ONE of the following ranks the various sites correctly in terms of plasma concentration of lidocaine? The site producing the highest plasma concentration is ranked first.

a) Brachial plexus, epidural, intercostal, caudal
b) Caudal, brachial plexus, intercostal, epidural
c) Epidural, intercostal, brachial plexus, caudal
d) Epidural, caudal, brachial plexus, intercostal
e) Intercostal, caudal, epidural, brachial plexus

Answer: e

Short explanation
In general, local anaesthetic is absorbed more rapidly from more vascular tissues, with intercostal block producing higher plasma levels than caudal, which in turn is higher than epidural, then brachial plexus blockade.

Long explanation
Along with dose administered, the main factor determining plasma concentration of local anaesthetic following infiltration for a nerve block is the vascularity of the surrounding tissues. Peak venous plasma concentration following a 100 mg dose of lidocaine is 1.5 µg/mL following an intercostal block. A caudal may produce a peak level of 1.2 µg/mL, an epidural 1.0 µg/mL and a brachial plexus block 0.6 µg/mL. This means that identical doses may be more toxic at different anatomical sites.

A plasma toxicity threshold for lidocaine is commonly quoted as 5.0 µg/mL. Inadvertent intravascular injection will rapidly achieve high plasma concentration and is of particular concern if the vessel into which the drug is injected supplies a major site of toxicity. For example, a dose of only 10 mg of lidocaine injected directly into the carotid or vertebral artery may cause seizures.

Other factors that may affect plasma concentration include the lipid profile of the tissues and the addition of other agents such as vasoconstrictors to the injectate.

Calvey N, Williams N. *Pharmacology for Anaesthetists*, 5th edn. Oxford: Blackwell, 2008; pp. 157–9.

SBA Question 81: Antidiuretic harmone

A farmer slips and falls in a remote field during a hot summer. He has nothing to eat and his only drink is whisky from a hip flask. He is not found for 3 days. On admission to hospital he is peripherally cold, with a heart rate of 110 beats/min and a blood pressure of 85/40 mmHg. Which of the following is the most potent stimulus for antidiuretic hormone release?

Answers:
a) Stimulation of central osmoreceptors
b) Stimulation of aortic arch baroreceptors
c) Ingestion of alcohol
d) Pain
e) Stress

Answer: b

Short explanation

Antidiuretic hormone (ADH) is also known as vasopressin. The main effects are potent vasoconstriction via V_1 receptors in arterioles and increasing renal collecting duct permeability to water by V_2 receptors on principal cells. The most potent stimulus to secretion is a drop in the circulating blood volume as detected by baroreceptors in the aortic arch and carotid sinus.

Long explanation

Antidiuretic hormone (ADH), also known as vasopressin, is a hormone synthesised in the hypothalamus and released from the posterior pituitary. It has two major effects. The first is to increase water permeability of the renal collecting ducts by action at V_2 receptors on the principal cells. This leads to an increase in reabsorption of water to maintain blood volume. The second effect is to cause vasoconstriction of the arterioles, increasing blood pressure. Other effects of ADH include promotion of platelet aggregation and the release of platelet factors, and increasing the amount of factor VIII released from endothelial cells.

Many factors increase release of ADH, including stress and pain, and an increase in osmolality as detected by osmoreceptors near the paraventricular nucleus and supraorbital nucleus in the hypothalamus – but the most potent stimulant of ADH is a drop in circulating blood volume as detected by baroreceptors in the carotid sinus and aortic arch. Alcohol reduces ADH secretion, causing polyuria.

There are various synthetic forms of ADH used therapeutically. Argipressin is a potent drug that can be used to reduce bleeding in oesophageal varices as well as to treat diabetes insipidus. Terlipressin is a prodrug metabolised into vasopressin, with a longer half-life. Desmopressin has less vasoconstrictor activity and is used to increase factor VIII levels in haemophilia and von Willebrand's disease.

Power I, Kam P. *Principles of Physiology for the Anaesthetist*. London: Arnold, 2001; p. 290.

SBA Question 82: Postoperative shivering

An adult patient distressed by shivering in the postoperative period would be most effectively treated with which ONE of the following?

a) Pethidine 25 mg
b) Doxapram 100 mg
c) Clonidine 150 μg

d) Ketanserin 10 mg
e) Alfentanil 250 μg

Answer: a

Short explanation

A systematic review in 2002 showed 25 mg of pethidine to be the most efficacious treatment for postoperative shivering.

Long explanation

Postoperative shivering is a problem that has been reported to affect from 5% to 60% of patients receiving general anaesthesia, and it may increase oxygen consumption by up to 500%.

A systematic review carried out by Kranke *et al.* in 2002 looked at 41 trials and eventually included 20 trials containing 1357 patients, of whom 944 received an active agent and 413 received a placebo. Of the 15 drugs used in the trials, the five used in this question had enough data to calculate efficacy statistics, including numbers needed to treat (NNT).

Pethidine was the superior agent for shivering at 1 minute, 5 minutes, 10 minutes and 15 minutes after treatment. At 5 minutes the NNTs were 1.3 for pethidine, 1.3 for clonidine, 1.7 for doxapram, 2.3 for ketanserin and 2.4 for alfentanil. At 10 minutes, pethidine had an NNT of 1.5, compared to 2.0 for clonidine. The combined data for the six trials involving pethidine showed no shivering at 5 minutes post-treatment in 133 out of 153 treated with pethidine compared to only 13 out of 147 in those given placebo.

Note that the question specifically asks for the agent that would be most effective, not what you would choose.

Kranke P, Eberhart LH, Roewer N, Tramer MR. Pharmacological treatment of post-operative shivering: a quantitative systematic review of randomized controlled trials. *Anesth Analg* 2002; **94**: 453–60. Available online at www.anesthesia-analgesia. org/content/94/2/453.full.pdf+html (accessed 15 March 2012).

SBA Question 83: Boiling point

A group of doctors from your hospital have recently returned from a charity trip climbing Mount Everest. They are relieved to be home as they said that they couldn't have a good cup of tea on the mountain. Which of these responses would best explain why?

a) The boiling point of water is 373.15 kelvin
b) The boiling point is the temperature of a substance at which its saturated vapour pressure equals external atmospheric pressure
c) A gas is a substance at a temperature above its critical temperature
d) Boiling point increases with increasing pressure
e) The saturated vapour pressure of a substance increases with increasing temperature

Answer: b

Short explanation

The boiling point of water at altitude is lower than at sea level, as the boiling point is the temperature of a substance at which its saturated vapour pressure equals external atmospheric pressure. Additional heat does not raise the temperature further, but provides the latent heat of vaporisation necessary for the liquid to evaporate. As the external atmospheric pressure is lower, the water will boil at a lower temperature, producing an inferior beverage. The boiling point of water at one atmosphere is 373.15 kelvin (K).

Long explanation

Temperature scales have been defined in the past by using known fixed temperatures, such as boiling and freezing points of water at one standard atmosphere pressure. The freezing point of water at sea level is 273.15 K (0 °C) and the boiling point is 373.15 K (100 °C). The transition of a substance between liquid and gas occurs at its boiling point. Changes in ambient pressure affect this point, and as the altitude increases and the pressure decreases, the temperature at which water boils will also decrease.

The term 'gas' is applied to a substance which is normally in its gaseous state at room temperature and atmospheric pressure. The critical temperature is the temperature above which a substance cannot be liquefied by pressure, regardless of its magnitude. A vapour is a gaseous substance below its critical temperature under ambient conditions.

The temperature of the transition between water and water vapour, its boiling point, will increase with increasing pressure, as discussed above. A vapour will form above a liquid by evaporation. At the point at which the vapour above the liquid is saturated, the pressure exerted by the vapour is said to be the saturated vapour pressure (SVP). It can also be defined as the pressure exerted by a vapour when in contact and in equilibrium with its liquid phase. The SVP of a liquid increases with increasing temperature. The boiling point is the temperature at which the SVP equals atmospheric pressure.

Smith T, Pinnock C, Lin T. *Fundamentals of Anaesthesia*, 3rd edn. Cambridge: Cambridge University Press, 2009; pp. 736–8.

SBA Question 84: Most important ventilatory stimulus

It is important to understand the physiological control of normal respiration. Considering a normal, unstressed, spontaneously respiring patient, which ONE of the following is considered to be most the important factor in regulating resting ventilation?

a) The effect of arterial oxygen tension at the central chemoreceptors
b) Changes in cerebrospinal fluid pH at the central chemoreceptors
c) The effect of arterial CO_2 tension at the peripheral chemoreceptors
d) Changes in plasma pH at peripheral chemoreceptors
e) The effect of arterial oxygen tension at the peripheral chemoreceptors

Answer: b

Short explanation

Arterial oxygen tension is only sensed by the peripheral chemoreceptors. The effect of pH and CO_2 at the peripheral chemoreceptors is not as significant as its effect on the central ones in controlling ventilation.

Long explanation

Control of breathing is complex and involves a number of receptors (chemoreceptors and lung receptors), central controllers (brainstem and cortex) and effectors to do the work (diaphragm and accessory muscles).

The most important stimulus for maintaining ventilation under normal conditions is the arterial tension of CO_2 ($PaCO_2$). The $PaCO_2$ is tightly regulated to within 0.5 kPa (3 mmHg) during rest and exercise (except severe exercise). The central chemoreceptors have a vital role in sensing the changes in arterial CO_2 tension and mediating the appropriate ventilatory response. The actual trigger for the chemoreceptors is H^+ ions. Changes in the concentration of H^+ are caused by the easy diffusion of CO_2 across the blood–brain barrier into the brain extracellular fluid. The barrier is relatively impermeable to charged particles, and therefore H^+ and bicarbonate do not easily diffuse across. Cerebrospinal fluid is slightly acidic compared with plasma. The increased CO_2 causes a shift in the equilibrium of the Henderson–Hasselbalch equation, which promotes the formation of H^+ and decreases the pH. It is this change in pH that mediates the appropriate increase in ventilation. An increase in the $PaCO_2$ stimulates ventilation, and the increase is fairly predictable. For each 0.1 kPa increase in $PaCO_2$ the alveolar ventilation increases by 1–2 L/min. The response to an increased $PaCO_2$ is augmented by hypoxia.

Compared with the central chemoreceptors, the peripheral chemoreceptors do not significantly contribute to the changes in ventilation secondary to an increase in CO_2 tension and H^+ ion concentration. However, it is thought that the peripheral chemoreceptors have a more rapid response to changes in CO_2 tension than the central ones.

Diagrams explaining control of breathing are available online at www.physiol.ox.ac.uk/ ~par/teaching/bm1_lect/lecture6.pdf (accessed 15 March 2012).

Kestin I. Control of breathing. *Update in Anaesthesia* 1992; **2**: article 1. Available online at www.nda.ox.ac.uk/wfsa/html/u02/u02_011.htm (accessed 15 March 2012).

West JB. *Respiratory Physiology*, 7th edn. Philadelphia, PA: Lippincott Williams & Wilkins, 2005; pp. 129–34.

SBA Question 85: Minimum inhibitory concentration

Minimum inhibitory concentration (MIC) may be used in the laboratory assessment of the efficacy of a particular antibiotic in the treatment of a particular organism. Which ONE of the following is the best definition of MIC?

a) MIC is the average plasma concentration caused by administering the lowest scheduled dose of an antibiotic

b) MIC is the lowest concentration of antibiotic required to kill 50% of bacterial colonies on a laboratory culture plate within 24 hours at standard temperature

c) MIC is the optimal concentration targeted for trough readings during therapeutic monitoring

d) MIC is the lowest concentration of an antimicrobial that will inhibit the visible growth of a microorganism after overnight incubation

e) MIC is the minimum antibiotic concentration in the plasma of adult humans required to cause a reduction in yield from blood cultures

Answer: d

Short explanation

MIC is a laboratory-derived value for the minimum concentration of an antimicrobial in a culture medium required to inhibit visible bacterial growth. It may (or may not) be used to determine minimum doses or trough levels, and may produce a reduction in bacteria in vivo.

Long explanation

Minimum inhibitary Concentration (MIC) is the most basic laboratory test of antimicrobial activity. It is the lowest concentration of an antimicrobial that will inhibit the visible growth of a microorganism after overnight incubation. Full details of the standardised method of determining MIC are available via the weblink below. MIC is of use when detecting resistance, when determining dosing schedules in antimicrobials with complex pharmacokinetics, or when looking at new antimicrobials, newly multi-resistant organisms and combinations of both.

Dosing schedules usually involve doses that will produce plasma concentrations a number of multiples of MIC, as the aim of therapy is to effectively and rapidly kill all bacteria before resistance can be developed. Trough levels may be above, at, or even below MIC for an agent that is therapeutically monitored, such as gentamicin. The main killing effect of this drug is caused by a high (8–10 times MIC) peak plasma concentration. A sub-MIC dose may still be effective, as the bacteria often have a 'memory' of the effect of gentamicin, which will therefore continue to work, despite sitting at low levels some of the time.

Andrews JM. Determination of minimum inhibitory concentration. *J Antimicrob Chemother* 2001; **48** (Suppl 1): 5–16. Available online at jac.oxfordjournals.org/content/48/suppl_1/5 (accessed 15 March 2012).

SBA Question 86: Antibiotic nephrotoxicity in the sick patient

A 68-year-old female is about to have an emergency laparotomy for suspected perforated colonic diverticulum. She looks unwell. She chronically has an eGFR of 33 mL/min/1.73 m^2 and weighs 80 kg. Which ONE of the following intravenous antibiotic regimens would you consider to be best in these circumstances?

a) Cefuroxime 1.5 g and metronidazole 500 mg
b) Gentamicin 240 mg and teicoplanin 800 mg
c) Vancomycin 1 g and gentamicin 160 mg
d) Tazocin 3.375 g
e) Gentamicin 160 mg, benzylpenicillin 1.8 g and metronidazole 500 mg

Answer: d

Short explanation
Tazocin is the best option presented here. It will provide the cover required for dirty lower gastrointestinal surgery with the lowest risk of significant renal toxicity.

Long explanation
This patient has perforated large bowel and stage III chronic kidney disease. She looks unwell and in light of her age and pathology is at high risk of developing sepsis and multi-organ dysfunction. She will need Gram-positive and Gram-negative cover with good anaerobic cover using an agent or agents with low nephrotoxicity. Nephrotoxic agents should therefore be avoided.

Gentamicin is nephrotoxic, as are, to a lesser extent, penicillins and cephalosporins. Gentamicin is particularly dangerous if the patient is dehydrated or hypotensive, which is likely in this case. Cephalosporins have been substantially phased out of UK prophylaxis regimens because of an increased risk of *Clostridium difficile* infection.

This only leaves the tazocin option, which is a good choice for a sick patient at risk of deteriorating renal dysfunction requiring cover for dirty lower gastrointestinal surgery. Normal adult dose is 4.5 g of tazocin (4 g of piperacillin and 0.5 g of tazobactam). In patients with an eGFR of 20–40 mL/min/1.73 m^2 the recommended dose is three-quarters the dose for a healthy adult.

SBA Question 87: Organophosphate poisoning

Ambulance control warns you that you are expecting a major incident in to your emergency department following exposure of eight people to a large dose of organophosphate (OP) insecticide. The patients have been decontaminated at the scene but are symptomatic of OP toxicity. Given the choice of a range of drug packs, which ONE would you choose?

a) Pack A contains diazepam, atropine, pralidoxime and ecothiopate
b) Pack B contains diazepam, atropine, suxamethonium and ecothiopate
c) Pack C contains diazepam, pralidoxime, suxamethonium and neostigmine
d) Pack D contains atropine, pralidoxime, suxamethonium and neostigmine
e) Pack E contains atropine, pralidoxime neostigmine and ecothiopate

Answer: a

Short explanation
Drugs of use in OP poisoning are the acetylcholinesterase reactivator pralidoxime, atropine to treat the muscarinic symptoms, and an anticonvulsant for seizure control.

Long explanation
Organophosphates (OPs) are common insecticides, and patients may present following accidental exposure or following an act of deliberate self-harm. The OPs are anticholinesterases, as they bind with a strong affinity to the esteratic site of acetylcholinesterase. Offset of action usually requires the body to synthesise new enzyme.

Primary treatment may include the administration of pralidoxime, which may reactivate phosphorylated acetylcholinesterase by promoting hydrolysis. Diazepam and atropine are of use in the symptomatic management of seizures and muscarinic manifestations, respectively. OPs also inhibit plasma butyrylcholinesterase. FFP has been given in the treatment of OP poisoning to selectively scavenge the OP onto the butyrylcholinesterase in the FFP, freeing up endogenous acetylcholinesterase. Ecothiopate is an OP that has been used in the management of glaucoma, where it relaxes the ciliary muscle, improving drainage. It should be discarded when pack A is opened. Suxamethonium should be used cautiously, as highly extended duration of block may occur due to inactive butyrylcholinesterase.

Peck T, Hill S, Williams M. *Pharmacology for Anaesthesia and Intensive Care*, 3rd edn. Cambridge: Cambridge University Press, 2008; pp. 195–6.

SBA Question 88: Measurement of V/Q mismatch

A patient with factor V Leiden deficiency presents with pleuritic pain and shortness of breath. Which ONE of the following tests would be most appropriate to investigate this patient for a pulmonary embolus?

a) Radioisotope scanning using xenon and technetium
b) Spirometry
c) Analysis of single-breath nitrogen washout
d) Radioisotope scanning using xenon and strontium
e) Lung function tests

Answer: a

Short explanation
Out of the tests offered, spirometry and lung function tests would not demonstrate a ventilation/perfusion abnormality. Analysis of single-breath nitrogen washout would not be quite appropriate because this measures anatomical dead space. Strontium is not used for radioisotope scanning.

Long explanation

There are a number of investigations that are used for pulmonary embolus (PE). After a thorough history and examination, blood and radiological investigations are considered. Blood tests include arterial blood gases and D-dimers (if low or moderate probability of PE). The type of imaging requested will depend on the facilities available.

The British Thoracic Society guidelines from 2003 recommend a CT pulmonary angiogram as the initial investigation after a chest radiograph for non-massive PE. For radioisotope scanning with xenon and technetium to be considered as the initial investigation a number of criteria must be met: facilities must be available on site, chest radiograph must be normal, there must be no significant cardiopulmonary disease, there must be standardised reporting, and a non-diagnostic test must be followed up with further imaging.

Ventilation/perfusion (V/Q) scans for PE are interpreted as normal or in terms of probabilities (high, intermediate, low or very low). If the scan is normal, the likelihood of clinically significant PE approaches zero. The degree of abnormality is based on the size and the number of mismatched or matched V/Q abnormalities. The radioisotope V/Q scan is conducted in two distinct parts. The ventilation study is performed by inhaling radioactive xenon-133, and images are then taken using a gamma camera. The perfusion study is conducted by injecting technetium-99-labelled albumin intravenously, and a further set of images is taken.

British Thoracic Society. British Thoracic Society guidelines for the management of suspected acute pulmonary embolism, 2003. *Thorax* 2003; **58**: 470–84. Available online at thorax.bmj.com/content/58/6/470 (accessed 15 March 2012).

SBA Question 89: Fetal circulation

The circulation of blood in the fetus differs from the adult circulation, and circulating blood has reduced oxygen saturations. In order of descending magnitude, order the following vessels according to their normal fetal saturations: umbilical artery (UA); umbilical vein (UV); superior vena cava (SVC); inferior vena cava (IVC); ductus venosus (DV); ductus arteriosus (DA).

a) UA, DV, IVC, UV, DA, SVC
b) UV, DV, IVC, DA, UA, SVC
c) UV, IVC, DV, UA, DA, SVC
d) UA, DV, IVC, SVC, DA, UV
e) UV, DV, IVC, SVC, DA, UA

Answer: b

Short explanation

Oxygen saturations in fetal vessels are as follows: umbilical vein (80%), ductus venosus (just less than 80%), IVC (67%), ductus arteriosus (60%), umbilical artery (45%), SVC (32%).

Long explanation

Fetal blood supply from the placenta is through the umbilical vein (sats approximately 80%) Flow is then divided, with 60% entering the ductus venosus (sats a little less than 80%) and the rest mixing with blood draining the gastrointestinal tract. The blood flows re-join in the IVC, reducing the overall sats to 65%, and thence the flow is to the right atrium (RA). Flow is again divided in the RA, with 60% directed across the foramen ovale to the left atrium/left ventricle to supply the head and the rest mixing with drainage from the head (from the SVC, which has very low sats of 32% due to a large oxygen extraction).

The result of mixing these bloods reduces saturations to around 60%. This blood is directed into the pulmonary artery, where the majority is directed across the ductus arteriosus (sats 60%) and into the aorta to supply the rest of the body and then return to the placenta via two umbilical arteries (sats 45%).

Thus, in order of magnitude: umbilical vein (80%), ductus venosus (just less than 80%), IVC (67%), ductus arteriosus (60%), umbilical artery (45%), SVC (32%).

Power I, Kam P. *Principles of Physiology for the Anaesthetist*. London: Arnold, 2001; pp. 356–7.

SBA Question 90: Oxygen carriage

A 38-year-old man smokes 40 cigarettes a day. An arterial blood gas taken in air shows him to have a PaO_2 of 95 mmHg, a $PaCO_2$ of 39 mmHg, a carboxyhaemoglobin (COHb) concentration of 6% and Hb of 13.5. Approximately where on the oxyhaemoglobin dissociation curve will his P_{50} be?

a) 5.3
b) 4.1
c) 3.8
d) 3.5
e) 2.9

Answer: e

Short explanation
The presence of carboxyhaemoglobin causes the oxyhaemoglobin dissociation curve to shift to the left, and therefore the P_{50} will be lower than a normal level of 3.5.

Long explanation
There is a direct relationship between the saturation of haemoglobin with oxygen and the partial pressure of oxygen in the blood. The higher the partial pressure the better saturated haemoglobin becomes. Plotting this relationship on a graph illustrates that it is not a linear relationship; the graph is a sigmoid shape. This relationship is explained by the physical characteristic of the haemoglobin protein. Adult haemoglobin has four chains (two α and two β), and these four chains can each bind one molecule of oxygen. Binding of oxygen is sequential: binding of one oxygen molecule induces a conformational change in protein chains that facilitates further oxygen binding, increasing affinity for the next molecule.

On the oxyhaemoglobin dissociation curve (ODC) there are three points that are of particular interest. The first point is the arterial point. This is the point on the graph representing arterial blood, where haemoglobin is close to 100% saturated at a partial pressure of oxygen of 13.5 kPa. The next point is the venous point, illustrating the venous blood, where the partial pressure of oxygen (breathing room air) is 5.3 kPa and haemoglobin is 75% saturated. The final point illustrates haemoglobin at 50% saturation. This is named the P_{50}, and it is an important point because it is used to define the position of the curve – that is, to describe if the curve is normal (with a P_{50} of 3.5 kPa) or if it has been shifted to the left or right. A variety of factors can shift the curve, and these determine if blood will bind more or less avidly to haemoglobin.

Factors such as carboxyhaemoglobin alter the rate at which oxygen is bound to and dissociated from haemoglobin. Carbon monoxide, like fetal haemoglobin, causes a leftward shift in the curve: with P_{50} less than 3.5 kPa, oxygen saturation is greater for any given partial pressure of oxygen. Acidosis, hypercarbia and 2,3-DPG all cause a rightward shift: oxygen saturation is less for any given partial pressure of oxygen, and oxygen dissociates to tissues more easily – for example at the peripheries, where more oxygen is thus available to cells.

Power I, Kam P. *Principles of Physiology for the Anaesthetist*. London: Arnold, 2001; pp. 69–71.

Paper 2

MTF Question 1: Postoperative prescribing

When prescribing in the postoperative period:

(a) Chronic pain analgesia should be stopped because of the risk of toxicity and interactions with acute pain analgesia
(b) Supplementary analgesia beyond codeine should be prescribed, as the efficacy of codeine varies hugely from individual to individual
(c) An antiemetic should be prescribed to all patients who have had a general anaesthetic
(d) A laxative such as lactulose should be prescribed to all elderly patients who have been prescribed postoperative opioids
(e) Unless contraindicated, paracetamol should be prescribed 'as required' for all patients

Answer: b,c

Short explanation
Chronic pain analgesia should be continued if possible. Lactulose is an expensive laxative and ispaghula husk would do just as well. Paracetamol should be prescribed regularly.

Long explanation
A stool bulking agent or faecal softener is an effective prophylactic agent against the constipation caused by opioids. It is good practice to prescribe such an agent to patients on opioids at risk of constipation, such as the elderly. The osmotic laxative lactulose is not substantially more effective in these circumstances and is considerably more expensive.

In general it is a good idea in patients experiencing even mild pain to keep a steady therapeutic plasma level of simple analgesic on board. At therapeutic doses, the low side-effect profile of paracetamol makes it the drug of choice. Steady levels are best maintained by having paracetamol prescribed for regular administration rather than on an 'as required' basis.

Patients having a general anaesthetic may have a risk of postoperative nausea and vomiting ranging from 5% to 80%. Even in the low-risk group, it is wise to prescribe an antiemetic for this unpleasant and debilitating adverse effect.

Codeine's analgesic effects come from it being metabolised to morphine and codeine-6-glucuronide. About 10% of Caucasians are unable to perform metabolism into morphine and find codeine to be a considerably less efficacious drug. It is therefore wise not to rely on codeine as the only prescribed postoperative analgesic.

If a patient is established on analgesics for a chronic condition it is recommended to keep the same dosing schedule into the postoperative period and then to add additional analgesia for acute pain on top of the background medication.

MTF Question 2: Environmental control of the operating theatre

With regard to the environmental control of the operating theatre, which of the following statements correctly describe passive scavenging systems?

(a) 33 mm tubing is used in the transfer system
(b) Volatile anaesthetic agents can be recirculated, saving money through conservation of use
(c) The use of nitrous oxide may reduce the efficiency of the system
(d) Atmospheric conditions may affect the cardiopulmonary status of the patient through the use of a passive scavenging system
(e) Atmospheric pollution is greater than with the active scavenging system

Answer: c,d

Short explanation

30 mm tubing is used in the transfer system. No recirculation of gas is possible from the scavenging system; the active and the passive both pass any waste gas to the atmosphere, polluting it to the same extent. Windy conditions or the use of a dense gas such as nitrous oxide may increase the forces required to expel waste gases through the passive system.

Long explanation

Scavenging refers to the method of extracting waste gases from the breathing system and venting them to an area where they will not be directly inhaled by staff or other patients. Scavenging systems can be classified as open or closed. Open refers to the basic system of extracting the gas from its point of entry into the theatre or anaesthetic room. Closed systems can be further subdivided into active and passive, and are a more commonly used method of waste gas removal in modern practice.

The passive scavenging system is a basic system of waste gas disposal where an exhaust port collects the waste gases from the expiratory valve of the breathing system or from the ventilator. The gases pass to the transfer system, which consists of 30 mm low-resistance tubing, and this conducts gases to the outside of the building, preferably above roof level where the risk of inhalation by others is minimised. An alternative solution is to pipe the waste gases to the exit port of the theatre ventilation system. Clearly this can only be used if the theatre air is not recirculated.

There are several disadvantages to the passive system. Firstly, the gases are pushed to the atmosphere solely by the expiratory power of the patient (remember that expiration is passive whether breathing spontaneously or if undergoing intermittent positive-pressure ventilation – IPPV). If the pathway to the atmosphere involves a vertical passage of gas, then the patient must overcome the atmospheric pressure required to push the gas over this distance. There may be significant forces to be overcome if the path to the atmosphere involves several floors of hospital. The forces may be compounded by the use of gases with higher density, such as nitrous oxide, or by adverse atmospheric conditions (such as high winds), which will further increase the forces required to expel waste gases. If these forces become excessive, adverse cardiopulmonary sequelae may be noted in relation to the higher intrapulmonary pressures.

No conservation of volatile agent is possible with either the active or the passive systems; conservation must occur within the anaesthetic breathing system itself, by the use of a circle system and low-flow anaesthesia. By the time gases are vented to the exhaust port, the final destination can only be the atmosphere. The quantity of waste gases released is also a factor of the flow rate and the breathing system used, so both the active and passive systems pollute the atmosphere to equal degrees.

Davis PD, Kenny GNC. *Basic Physics and Measurement in Anaesthesia*, 5th edn. Oxford: Butterworth–Heinemann, 2003; pp. 237–52.

MTF Question 3: Ion channels

Which of the following statements about ion channels are correct?

(a) Voltage-gated ion channels can be either open or closed
(b) The binding site of a ligand-gated ion channel is usually in the extracellular domain
(c) The β_2-adrenoreceptor is an example of a ligand-gated ion channel
(d) The duration of opening of voltage-gated channels is purely controlled by the membrane potential of the cell
(e) The NMDA glutamate receptor exhibits both voltage-gated and ligand-gated activation

Answer: b,e

Short explanation

Voltage-gated sodium channels also have an inactive state. Adrenoreceptors are metabotropic (i.e. G-protein-coupled) receptors and are not directly linked to an ion channel. Endogenous and exogenous modulators influence voltage-gated channels. NMDA receptors can 'add' signals, and this plays a role in synaptic plasticity.

Long explanation

Broadly speaking, ion channels are opened through one of two different mechanisms: they are either voltage-gated or ligand-gated.

Voltage-gated channels are transmembrane proteins with a central ion pore that can exist in several states. The best-studied is the sodium channel, which can be closed, open or inactive (refractory). As the membrane becomes more depolarised a threshold is reached, at which point the central ion channel opens, allowing the passage of sodium ions into the cell down their concentration gradient and depolarising the cell further. This leads to a positive-feedback loop and a rapid spike in membrane potential, opening further sodium channels (an action potential). After a period of approximately 0.7 ms the channel becomes inactivated, probably by the movement of part of the intracellular protein into the pore, and it then remains refractory for several milliseconds before it again takes up the closed conformation, ready for a new action potential. Modulatory proteins and other factors in the cell membrane or within the cell, as well as exogenous factors such as local anaesthetic drugs, influence the frequency and duration of opening of voltage-gated channels. This is seen with all voltage-gated channels, but it seems to be most important to potassium and calcium voltage-gated channel activity.

Ligand-gated ion channels are proteins consisting of a central ion pore with a ligand-binding site (usually) in the extracellular domain. They include ionotropic neurotransmitter receptor molecules such as the nicotinic acetylcholine receptor, the GABA$_A$ and glycine receptors, and the AMPA and NMDA glutamate receptors. Binding of the ligand (e.g. acetylcholine, GABA) causes the ion pore to open, again allowing ions to flow down their concentration gradient. As with the voltage-gated ion channels, modulator proteins and other factors can influence the activity of these receptors, and many drugs modify these receptors in this way (e.g. benzodiazepines increase the frequency of GABA binding at the $GABA_A$ receptor). NMDA receptors are a special case since they respond to both ligand and voltage signals: it is suggested that their ability to increase the responsiveness of synapses underlies learning and memory.

Power I, Kam P. *Principles of Physiology for the Anaesthetist*, 2nd edn. London: Hodder, 2007.

MTF Question 4: Parasympathetic nervous system

Regarding the parasympathetic nervous system:

(a) Cranial nerves III, VII, VIII and X carry parasympathetic afferent fibres to the pupil and salivary glands
(b) Sacral outflow originates from the 2nd, 3rd and 4th sacral segments of the spinal cord
(c) The vagus nerve innervates the ureter
(d) Bronchial muscle constriction is mediated via thoracic fibres
(e) Sacral fibres innervate the distal colon, rectum, bladder and reproductive organs

Answer: b,c,e

Short explanation
Cranial nerves III, VII, IX and X carry parasympathetic fibres. There is no thoracic outflow component to the parasympathetic nervous system.

Long explanation
The parasympathetic nervous system is primarily responsible for regulation of bodily functions while the body is at rest. Some of these functions include lacrimation, salivation, urination, digestion and defecation. The parasympathetic nervous system is described as having a craniosacral outflow. The cranial nerves that carry parasympathetic outflow are the oculomotor nerve, the facial nerve, the glossopharyngeal nerve and the vagus nerve. The parasympathetic nerves that arise from the 2nd, 3rd and 4th sacral nerves are also called the pelvic splanchnic nerves. Approximately two-thirds of all parasympathetic fibres are carried in the two vagus nerves. The preganglionic fibres of the parasympathetic outflow are long, and the postganglionic fibres are short.

Bakewell S. The autonomic nervous system. *Update in Anaesthesia* 1995; (**5**): article 6. Available online at www.nda.ox.ac.uk/wfsa/html/u05/u05_010.htm (accessed 15 March 2012).

MTF Question 5: Cardiovascular changes in pregnancy

Regarding the cardiovascular changes associated with pregnancy:

(a) Significant cardiovascular changes can be observed by week 8 gestation
(b) Heart rate increases most in the third trimester
(c) Aortocaval compression typically becomes a problem around 16 weeks
(d) A 10–15 mmHg rise in mean arterial pressure is typical
(e) Cardiac output returns to pre-pregnancy levels by 48 hours postpartum

Answer: a

Short explanation
During pregnancy, heart rate increases most in the first trimester. It would be exceptionally unusual for aortocaval compression to occur before 20 weeks. Progressive vasodilation offsets the rise in cardiac output, obtunding any potential

rise in arterial pressure. Cardiac output returns to pre-pregnancy levels by 2 weeks post-partum.

Long explanation

During pregnancy, the maternal cardiovascular system must facilitate increased uteroplacental flow (about 750 mL/min at term) and substrate delivery to the fetus. The hormones elevated in order to maintain the pregnancy result in changes in maternal physiology and have significant effects on the cardiovascular system. Progesterone and prostaglandins cause a smooth muscle relaxation that is manifest as a vasodilation and reduction of systemic vascular resistance (by 30% during the first trimester).

Via oestrogens stimulating the renin–angiotensin–aldosterone system, inducing salt and water retention, blood volume progressively increases throughout pregnancy. This increased preload increases stroke volume so that, in combination with a 25% increase in heart rate (most of which occurs in the first trimester), cardiac output is increased by 50%. Despite this, any potential consequent rise in arterial blood pressure is obtunded by the vasodilation, such that a modest decrease in systolic and diastolic blood pressure is typically seen. The distribution of this elevated cardiac output is to the uteroplacental circulation (up to 850 mL/min at term), the kidneys, breasts, skin and gut.

The supine hypotension syndrome occurs when the pregnant woman is supine and the gravid uterus concurrently compresses the aorta and the inferior vena cava. This produces an acute rise in afterload and a reduction in preload (as venous return is decreased), resulting in a sudden drop of cardiac output. The subject may complain of light-headedness or nausea as a result or be intrinsically reluctant to adopt that position. For this to occur, the pelvic mass (which need not necessarily be a gravid uterus) must be of sufficient volume to compress the great vessels. Although there are case reports of this occurring as early as 20 weeks gestation, it would be unlikely at 16 weeks.

Although times quoted vary, the time taken for return of cardiac output to pre-pregnancy levels is of the order of 2 weeks.

MTF Question 6: Vomiting centre afferents

Regarding vomiting centre afferents:

(a) The mechano- and chemoreceptors in the gastrointestinal tract are both vagal nerve afferents
(b) The vomiting centre is a discrete area of reticular formation in the medulla
(c) The vomiting centre receives afferent fibres from cranial nerves V, VII, IX, X and XII
(d) Cranial nerve X is the predominant afferent input from the heart
(e) Raised intracranial pressure on the third ventricle stimulates vomiting

Answer: a,d

Short explanation

The vomiting centre is a group of complex neuronal interconnections. Motor efferent fibres travel via cranial nerves V, VII, IX, X and XII. Raised intracranial pressure on the floor of the fourth ventricle stimulates vomiting.

Long explanation

The vomiting centre (VC) is found in the dorsolateral reticular formation in the medulla, and rather than being a discrete control centre it consists of a group of complex interconnections between the different central control centres involved in the vomiting reflex.

The vomiting centre receives afferent inputs from many areas of the body. The gastrointestinal tract has mechanoreceptors that detect intraluminal pressure changes and chemoreceptors that detect intraluminal environmental changes. The chemoreceptors detect acid–alkaline changes, chemical irritants and bacterial endo- and exotoxins. Both the mechano- and chemoreceptors are linked to vagal afferents which send impulses to the VC.

The VC also receives afferents from the heart, the peritoneum and abdominal organs. As in the gastrointestinal tract, these are vagal afferents transmitted by the vagus nerve (cranial nerve X). The afferent impulses from the heart are predominantly vagal.

The vestibular apparatus (motion effects), chemoreceptor trigger zone (neurotransmitters and drugs) and higher centres all contribute afferent inputs to the VC. Raised intracranial pressure on the floor of the fourth ventricle stimulates vomiting; the third ventricle is not known to have this effect. These afferents are processed in the VC, and coordinated motor efferents, via cranial nerves V, VII, IX, X and XII, result in the vomiting reflex.

Smith T, Pinnock C, Lin T. *Fundamentals of Anaesthesia*, 3rd edn. Cambridge: Cambridge University Press, 2009; pp. 446–7.
Yentis S, Hirsch N, Smith G. *Anaesthesia and Intensive Care A–Z: an Encyclopaedia of Principles and Practice*, 3rd edn. Edinburgh: Butterworth–Heinemann, 2004; p. 542.

MTF Question 7: Epidural analgesia in labour

Regarding the use of epidural analgesia with low-dose bupivacaine and fentanyl in labour:

(a) Epidural analgesia produces a reduced Apgar score at 1 minute but not at 5 minutes
(b) Women receiving an epidural are more likely to have a forceps or vacuum delivery
(c) Epidural analgesia increases the risk of a caesarean section
(d) The siting of an epidural increases the likelihood of long-term postpartum backache
(e) It is not uncommon for women receiving an epidural to have a significant rise in body temperature

Answer: b,e

Short explanation
The current body of research evidence would indicate that epidural analgesia does not affect Apgar scores, the likelihood of requiring a caesarean section or the incidence of long-term postpartum back pain.

Long explanation
Concern has been expressed for many years that epidural analgesia in labour is a cause of an increased likelihood of requiring a caesarean section. Systematic review has failed to demonstrate such an effect.

Epidural analgesia has been associated with lengthening of the second stage of labour and a higher rate of forceps or vacuum delivery. This is an association rather than a causation. The requirement for an epidural may purely be a marker of a more complex labour, increasing the likelihood of an assisted delivery. Trials have failed to demonstrate an increase in the rate of chronic backache postpartum. Epidural analgesia does not affect Apgar scores (at either 1 or 5 minutes) and there is some evidence that epidurals improve fetal acid–base status.

Some women receiving epidurals in labour have been found to have a significant rise in temperature. The mechanism and impact of this 'epidural fever' are unclear. Suggested contributory factors include the cessation of hyperventilation, an increase in shivering and a decrease in sweating. This temperature rise is contrary to the general temperature effect found in general surgery with epidural blockade when uncontrolled vasodilation leads to additional heat loss.

National Collaborating Center for Women's and Children's Health. *Intrapartum Care*. NICE clinical guideline, September 2007. Available online at www.gserve.nice.org. uk/nicemedia/pdf/IntrapartumCareSeptember2007mainguideline.pdf (accessed 15 March 2012).

MTF Question 8: Statistical power

Which of the following will reduce the power of statistical analysis?

(a) Increasing the sample size
(b) Decreasing the significance level
(c) Increasing the probability of a type two (beta) error
(d) Increasing the probability of a type one (alpha) error
(e) Decreasing the magnitude of the effect of the treatment intervention

Answer: b

Short explanation

The power of statistical analysis is the probability of NOT committing a type 2 (beta) error (i.e. 1 – B, where B is the beta or type 2 error). Power of statistical analysis increases as sample size increases, effect size increases and significance level increases.

Long explanation

Lack of adequate power in statistical analysis is a prime culprit in erroneous interpretation of data, and as a result carrying out a power analysis early in the design stage of a research project is usually highly desirable. The power of statistical analysis is the probability of NOT committing a type 2 (beta) error, where a type 2 error is defined as the failure to reject an erroneous null hypothesis (i.e. 1 – B, where B is the beta or type 2 error).

There are three main factors that influence the power of any statistical analysis:

- the sample size
- the effect size
- the significance level (or the probability that the observed difference in the results is due to chance)

The sample size will determine the amount of sampling error inherent in any test result. The larger the sample size (as a proportion of the total population being examined), the lower the sampling error and therefore the power of any statistical analysis will be greater.

The effect size is, in essence, the difference between outcomes in the two populations being examined. The greater the effect size (i.e. the greater the difference between the populations being examined), the greater the power of any statistical analysis on the data being examined.

The significance level is an assessment of how unlikely a result must be, if the null hypothesis is true, to be considered significant. This is your $p < 0.05$, $p < 0.01$, etc. seen in the statistical analysis of data. The higher the significance level set, the greater the power of a statistical analysis. If you increase the significance (decrease the p value) then you are more likely to reject the null hypothesis. Therefore one is less likely to accept the null hypothesis when it is false (less likely to make a type 2 error), so the power of the statistical analysis will increase.

Other factors that may have an effect on the power of an analysis include the design of the study and the precision with which data are obtained.

MTF Question 9: The effects of renal failure

Which of the following statements about the pharmacological effects of renal failure are correct?

(a) Vecuronium should be avoided in patients with acute kidney injury (AKI)
(b) Patients with renal failure may require a higher loading dose of a drug in order to achieve a therapeutic plasma concentration
(c) Dose reductions can be calculated by multiplying the usual dose by the ratio of the patient's creatinine clearance and a normal creatinine clearance
(d) The targeted plasma concentration of a drug will be the same in renal failure as in a healthy patient
(e) Renal failure causes accumulation of propofol and prolongs the effect of propofol infusion

Answer: a,b,c,d

Short explanation
Vecuronium is largely excreted unchanged by the kidney. Renal failure can cause an increased volume of distribution, necessitating a higher loading dose. Dose in renal failure = usual dose × (current creatinine clearance / normal creatinine clearance). Propofol is metabolised in the liver and does not accumulate in renal failure.

Long explanation
Renal failure has numerous implications for pharmacokinetics. Most obviously, drugs that are usually renally excreted may accumulate in the body. The severity of this effect depends on the drug's dependence on renal excretion: a drug which is excreted 100% unchanged in the urine may have a markedly prolonged duration of action. The drugs most likely to encounter this problem in anaesthesia are the aminosteroid non-depolarising muscle relaxants vecuronium and rocuronium, although the use of sugam-madex to reverse their activity may allow them to be used in some cases.

Some drugs are metabolised in the kidney itself, and this process can also be affected by renal failure. In addition, renal failure (especially chronic kidney disease, CKD) often leads to fluid retention and a consequent increase in total body water and hence apparent volume of distribution. Targeted plasma drug concentrations are the same as for a healthy patient, but if the volume of distribution is increased this implies that a higher loading dose may be required to produce this concentration.

Since clearance is likely to be reduced, the rate of decline of the drug concentration will be slowed. For this reason a longer interval may be required between drug doses. In general terms, if the patient's creatinine clearance is known then the dose required (D) can be calculated from the equation D = usual dose × (patient's creatinine clearance / normal creatinine clearance). When calculating drug regimes for patients with renal failure all these factors must be borne in mind.

Peck T, Hill S, Williams M. *Pharmacology for Anaesthesia and Intensive Care*, 3rd edn. Cambridge: Cambridge University Press, 2008.

MTF Question 10: Mechanism of action of NSAIDs

Regarding the mechanism of action of non-steroidal anti-inflammatory drugs (NSAIDs):

(a) They inhibit the enzymes cyclooxygenase and lipoxygenase in the metabolism of arachidonic acid
(b) Their antipyretic activity is brought about via reduced production of PGE_2
(c) Increased levels of leukotrienes are as a result of increased activity of lipoxygenase
(d) Production of phospholipase A_2 is reduced
(e) Platelet production of prostacyclin is inhibited

Answer: b,c

Short explanation
NSAIDs inhibit cyclooxygenase, which metabolises arachidonic acid. Phospholipase A_2 is inhibited by steroids. Prostacyclin (PGI_2) is produced by the vascular endothelium.

Long explanation
Non-steroidal anti-inflammatory drugs (NASIDs) are used throughout all areas of modern clinical medicine. The main beneficial activities of these drugs are their anti-inflammatory, antipyretic and antiplatelet activities. These effects are mediated through inhibition of enzymes involved in the metabolism of arachidonic acid and the production of inflammatory mediators. Arachidonic acid is a product of membrane phospholipid breakdown. Arachidonic acid is metabolised by cyclooxygenase to cyclic endoperoxidases and by lipoxygenase to leukotrienes. Cyclic endoperoxidases then lead to the formation of prostaglandins, prostacyclin (via the vascular endothelium) and thromboxane A_2 (via platelets).

NSAIDs inhibit the activity of cyclooxygenase, leading to reduced production of these mediators. Prostaglandins such as PGE_2 and $PGF_{2\alpha}$ usually cause fever via stimulation of the hypothalamic thermoregulatory centres. Prostacyclin promotes vasodilation and inhibits platelet aggregation. Thromboxane is produced by platelets in response to collagen exposure and tissue damage, and promotes vasoconstriction and platelet aggregation.

Inhibition of cyclooxygenase by NSAIDs is irreversible. In the context of platelet cyclooxygenase this remains inactive for the lifepan of the platelet, as the platelet has no ability to regenerate cyclooxygenase. The vascular endothelium can regenerate cyclooxygenase and allow further production of prostacyclin. When cyclooxygenase is inhibited, the metabolism of arachidonic acid to leukotrienes can still occur. In some circumstances the activity of lipoxygenase may be increased, leading to more leukotrienes being produced.

Good diagrams and explanations can be found at www.arthritis.co.za/arachid.html (accessed 15 March 2012).

MTF Question 11: Catecholamine synthesis

Which of the following statements regarding catecholamine synthesis and metabolism are correct?

(a) Tyrosine is converted from phenylalanine by decarboxylation
(b) Dopamine is the first catecholamine formed through the synthetic pathway
(c) Tyrosine hydroxylase facilitates the rate-limiting step
(d) Noradrenaline is converted to adrenaline by the enzyme catechol-O-methyltransferase
(e) Monoamine oxidase is involved in the metabolism of catecholamines

Answer: b,c,e

Short explanation
Catecholamine synthesis begins with the hydroxylation of phenylalanine to tyrosine. The following step, hydroxylation of tyrosine to dihydroxyphenylalanine (DOPA), is rate-limiting. The final conversion of noradrenaline to adrenaline is catalysed by phenylethanolamine N-methyltransferase (PNMT).

Long explanation

Catecholamines are hormones primarily synthesised in and secreted from the adrenal medulla. They are compounds containing a catechol (a benzene ring with hydroxide groups at positions 3 and 4) and amine groups. Catecholamines can be naturally occurring (dopamine, noradrenaline, adrenaline) or synthetic (isoprenaline, dobutamine). Synthesis of the naturally occurring catecholamines proceeds through a step-wise process. L-tyrosine may be derived from the diet or through hydroxylation of phenylalanine in the liver.

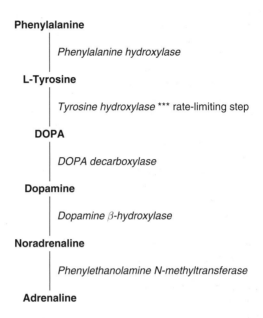

The formation of dihydroxyphenylalanine (DOPA) and dopamine occurs in the cytoplasm of cells of the adrenal medulla. Dopamine is transported into chromaffin cells by an active process where it is converted to noradrenaline. In approximately 80% of chromaffin cells, noradrenaline is subsequently converted to adrenaline.

The half-life of circulating catecholamines is between 10 and 30 seconds. This rapid termination is secondary to two processes, uptake of catecholamines into tissue and sympathetic nerve endings or enzymatic metabolism. Catechol-O-methyltransferase is an extraneuronal enzyme found primarily in the liver and kidneys. This enzyme catalyses the metabolism of adrenaline or noradrenaline to metadrenaline and normetadrenaline respectively. Monoamine oxidase is the enzyme responsible for the converstion of (nor)metadrenaline to vanillylmandelic acid (VMA), which is excreted in the urine.

Power I, Kam P. *Principles of Physiology for the Anaesthetist*. London: Arnold, 2001; pp. 304–6.

Yentis S, Hirsch N, Smith G. *Anaesthesia and Intensive Care A–Z: an Encyclopaedia of Principles and Practice*, 3rd edn. Edinburgh: Butterworth-Heinemann, 2004; p. 102.

MTF Question 12: P_{50}

The P_{50}:

(a) Is the arterial oxygen tension at which haemoglobin saturation is 50%
(b) Moves to the right according to the Bohr effect

(c) Is typically less than 3.5 kPa in the presence of carbon monoxide poisoning
(d) Represents the haemoglobin saturation when arterial oxygen tension is 50 mmHg
(e) Shifts to the left in fetal blood

Answer: a,b,c,e

Short explanation

The P_{50} is the point on the x axis of the oxyhaemoglobin dissociation curve (arterial oxygen tension) where haemoglobin saturation is 50%. The normal value is 3.5 kPa (27 mmHg). A P_{50} less than this value constitutes a leftwards shift of the curve, as seen in carbon monoxide poisoning and fetal blood.

Long explanation

The oxyhaemoglobin dissociation curve (ODC) is a plot of oxygen saturation of haemoglobin versus arterial oxygen tension for normal adult haemoglobin and partial pressure of carbon dioxide at 37 °C. The P_{50} is an important point on the ODC which enables comparison between curves in differing conditions. It is defined as the partial pressure of oxygen at which haemoglobin saturation is 50%. The normal value is approximately 3.5 kPa (27 mmHg). This point is most commonly used to describe the position of the ODC as it lies on the steepest part of the curve. The position of the ODC can be affected by the following factors:

	Leftwards shift	Rightwards shift
$[H^+]$	↓	↑
Temperature	↓	↑
$PaCO_2$	↓	↑
2,3-DPG	↓	↑
Anaemia		✓
Carbon monoxide	✓	
HbF	✓	
HbS		✓
Methaemoglobin	✓	

The shift refers to the position of the P_{50}. A rightwards shift represents a reduction in the affinity of haemoglobin for oxygen, and haemoglobin saturation is lower for a given partial pressure of oxygen. Conversely, a leftward shift represents an increased affinity of haemoglobin for oxygen, thereby favouring oxygen binding. The Bohr effect describes a rightwards shift in the ODC associated with hypercapnia and/or acidosis. This results in the unloading of oxygen in the tissues where carbon dioxide levels are high.

Yentis S, Hirsch N, Smith G. *Anaesthesia and Intensive Care A–Z: an Encyclopaedia of Principles and Practice*, 3rd edn. Edinburgh: Butterworth–Heinemann, 2004; pp. 68, 393.

MTF Question 13: Systole

Regarding the cardiac cycle in a healthy adult:

(a) In a healthy heart coronary perfusion to both ventricles occurs primarily during diastole

(b) During systole, the aortic valve opens at approximately 120 mmHg, reflecting the systolic blood pressure
(c) The dicrotic notch marks the end of systole
(d) The right ventricle reaches maximum pressures of 25 mmHg during systole
(e) During systole, the pressure gradient between left ventricle and aorta is less than 5 mmHg

Answer: c,d,e

Short explanation
Coronary perfusion of the left ventricle occurs mainly during diastole, when the myocardium is relaxed and the subendocardial vessels are patent. In contrast, the right ventricle is perfused during both diastole and systole, as intraventricular and intramural pressures are low. After the aortic valve opens, the pressure within the system will continue to rise, peaking at systolic pressure.

Long explanation
The cardiac cycle in a normal adult heart is intuitive if approached in a systematic manner. As this question focuses on systolic function, so will this explanation.

Systole begins with the closure of the mitral and tricuspid valves. At this stage, the aortic and pulmonary valves are also closed. During this period of isovolumetric contraction, the ventricle contracts against closed valves and the intraventricular pressure rises. When the intraventricular pressure exceeds pressure in the aorta and pulmonary artery, the semilunar valves open and ejection begins. Initially, the intra-ventricular pressure continues to rise during ejection, to reach a maximum pressure of 120 mmHg and 25 mmHg for the left and right ventricles respectively. As ventricular pressure falls below that in the aorta and pulmonary valves, the semilunar valves close. The dicrotic notch represents the closure of the aortic valve and the subsequent elastic recoil of the aorta, which leads to a transient rise in aortic pressure. This downward deflection illustrates the end of systole.

The diastolic blood pressure is the minimum pressure in the aorta immediately preceding ejection of blood from the left ventricle, and it is due to the distribution of blood into the systemic circulation. The systolic blood pressure is the maximum pressure reached in the aorta and left ventricle during systole. During ejection, the pressure waveforms of the left ventricle and aorta are very similar, differing by a gradient of only 1–2 mmHg.

Smith T, Pinnock C, Lin T. *Fundamentals of Anaesthesia*, 3rd edn. Cambridge: Cambridge University Press, 2009; pp. 279–81.

MTF Question 14: Opioid receptors

Which of the following are true regarding opioid receptors?

(a) All opioid receptors are ionotropic
(b) All opioid receptors are metabotropic
(c) The opioid receptors are coupled to Gs proteins
(d) There are four classical opioid receptors
(e) Ketocyclazacine is an antagonist at all endogenous opioid receptors

Answer: b

Short explanation

Opioid receptors are metabotropic, not ionotropic, as they are associated with G proteins, and are of the Gi subgroup. There are three classical receptors (DOP, KOP, MOP) and one non-classical receptor (NOP). Ketocyclazacine is the original agonist at the KOP receptor but exerts some antagonist effects at the MOP receptor.

Long explanation

The opioid receptors are metabotropic, as they are G-protein-coupled. Binding of a ligand to the extracellular surface of the receptor causes a conformational change and coupling of the G protein subunits, activating intermediate messengers. Ligands binding to ionotropic receptors cause a change in membrane ion permeability (e.g. the nicotinic acetylcholine receptor at the neuromuscular junction).

Opioid receptors are linked to inhibitory Gi proteins; activation of the receptor causes closure of voltage-sensitive calcium channels and cell membrane hyperpolarisation, and prevention of nerve transmission.

The opioid receptors are named according to the International Union of Basic and Clinical Pharmacology (IUPHAR) as DOP, KOP, MOP (classical receptors) and NOP (non-classical receptor); this nomeclature is based on the original ligand found to bind to the receptor MOP (μ, morphine), KOP (κ, ketocyclazacine), DOP (δ, vas deferens; receptor first found in the mouse vas deferens), NOP (nociceptin/orphanin FQ). The OP1 (DOP), OP2 (KOP), OP3 (MOP), OP4 (NOP) nomenclature was based on the order in which the receptors were cloned.

Ketocyclazacine is the original agonist at the KOP receptor, but it has some antagonist effects at the MOP receptor that limit its clinical use.

Peck T, Hill S, Williams M. *Pharmacology for Anaesthesia and Intensive Care*, 3rd edn. Cambridge: Cambridge University Press, 2008.

MTF Question 15: Control of blood volume

Which of the following statements regarding the control of blood volume are correct?

(a) Low-pressure baroreceptors are located in the carotid sinus
(b) The juxtaglomerular apparatus releases angiotensinogen in response to sympathetic activity
(c) The arterial baroreceptor reflex transmits signals to higher centres via the glossopharyngeal nerve
(d) The thirst sensation is partially mediated by antidiuretic hormone
(e) Long-term control includes redistribution of blood from reservoirs

Answer: c,d

Short explanation

Carotid sinus baroreceptors are high pressure, with the low-pressure receptors in sites such as the atria. The juxtaglomerular apparatus releases renin in response to sympathetic activity which acts on angiotensinogen, an α_2-globulin mainly secreted by the liver and present in the circulation. Short-term control of blood volume involves redistribution of blood, and longer-term control involves the balance between fluid intake and excretion.

Long explanation

Blood volume control can be thought of as an afferent limb, a central control system and efferent mechanisms. The afferent limb largely relies upon the baroreceptors, which can be divided into low- and high-pressure receptors as well as intrarenal baroreceptors.

The low-pressure baroreceptors are venous stretch receptors located in the atria, left ventricle, roots of the great veins, and pulmonary vascular bed. They are largely involved in the control of blood volume.

The high-pressure baroreceptors are arterial stretch receptors. They are present in the carotid sinus and aortic arch and, when stimulated, transmit signals to the vasomotor centres in the medulla via the glossopharyngeal and vagus nerves respectively. The baroreceptor reflex is a negative feedback mechanism that employs these high-pressure baroreceptors. When stimulated in response to stretch, impulse firing frequency increases. This leads to an inhibition of sympathetic activity in the pressor centre of the medulla and activates the cardioinhibitory centres.

The intrarenal baroreceptors are housed within the juxtaglomerular apparatus. Renal sympathetic stimulation results in renal vasoconstriction upstream of the granular renin-containing cells. Because of an increase in vascular resistance, arteriolar wall tension is decreased, which is sensed by baroreceptors present in the afferent arteriole. This is one of the mechanisms that stimulate renin release. A decrease in extracellular volume will have the same effect, working via the afferent arteriolar baroreceptor reflex.

The thirst centre is located in the hypothalamus. The sensation of thirst is mediated by angiotensin II, hypothalamic osmoreceptors and low-pressure stretch receptors. Activation of thirst leads to a behavioural change as the individual seeks hydration, as well as a release of vasopressin (antidiuretic hormone, ADH) from the posterior pituitary to minimise fluid excretion. The release of vasopressin also partially mediates the thirst sensation.

Power I, Kam P. *Principles of Physiology for the Anaesthetist*. London: Arnold, 2001; pp. 72–3.
Smith T, Pinnock C, Lin T. *Fundamentals of Anaesthesia*, 3rd edn. Cambridge: Cambridge University Press, 2009; pp. 312–15, 410–11.

MTF Question 16: Neurotransmitter receptor matching

Which of the following combinations correctly describes a neurotransmitter (stated first) matched with the receptor at which it is an agonist (stated second)?

(a) α-Amino-3-hydroxy-5-methyl-4-isoxazole-propionate (AMPA) and *N*-methyl-D-aspartate (NMDA)
(b) Substance P and neurokinin 1
(c) Glutamate and γ-aminobutyric acid A ($GABA_A$)
(d) Glycine and NMDA
(e) Kainate and glutamate

Answer: b

Short explanation

AMPA and kainate are receptors (not endogenous neurotransmitters), both stimulated by glutamate. GABA agonises GABA receptors. Glycine is a co-agonist at the NMDA receptor but not an agonist.

Long explanation

Glutamate is an excitatory amino acid neurotransmitter that may act at the NMDA, AMPA, kainate or metabotropic glutamate receptor. These synapses are involved in transmission of nociception, central sensitisation and the 'wind-up' phenomenon. Kainate is an exogenous molecule derived from red algae and found to stimulate the kainate receptor. AMPA is an artificial glutamate analogue. Neither AMPA nor kainate are neurotransmitters. The agonism of NMDA receptors by glutamate is antagonised by the drug ketamine. Substance P and neurokinin A are also involved in pain pathways and are peptide neurotransmitters that both stimulate neurokinin-1 receptors. Glycine is an inhibitory neurotransmitter confined to the central nervous system and acts at glycine recptors. It is also a co-agonist with glutamate at the NMDA receptor but is not an agonist when acting alone.

Gamma-aminobutyric acid A ($GABA_A$) and $GABA_B$ are receptors at which GABA is an agonist, not glutamate. The β subunit of $GABA_A$ is potentiated by thiobarbiturates. The α subunit of $GABA_A$ appears to be the binding site of benzodiazepines. The $GABA_A$ receptor is a ligand-gated ionotropic Cl^- channel. The $GABA_B$ receptor is metabotropic.

MTF Question 17: Osmolality

Which of the following statements concerning osmolality are true?

(a) Plasma osmolality ranges from 280 to 295 mOsm/L
(b) Osmolality of body fluid is usually higher than its osmolarity
(c) Antidiuretic hormone is secreted in response to a drop in osmolality
(d) Osmolality is maintained constant throughout the body compartments
(e) Osmolality is regulated by osmoreceptors located in the brainstem

Answer: b,d

Short explanation
Osmolality of body fluid is usually higher than its osmolarity because of protein and lipid content. Plasma osmolality is 280–295 mOsm/kg. Osmolality is regulated by osmoreceptors located outside the blood–brain barrier in the hypothalamus. These receptors stimulate a release of antidiuretic hormone.

Long explanation
Osmolality is defined as the concentration of a solution expressed as osmoles of solute per kilogram of solvent. Units include Osm/kg H_2O or mOsm/kg H_2O.

Osmolarity is the concentration of a solution expressed in osmoles of solute per litre of solution. Units include Osm/L or mOsm/L.

Osmolality of body fluid is usually higher than its osmolarity because of protein and lipid content, which occupy a small but finite volume. Due to the high molecular weights of proteins and lipids, they occupy more space within a solution. Therefore, if you were to take 1 kg of solvent, such as water, there will be more osmoles of fat and protein in the solution than the number of osmoles in 1 L of the same solution. Thus, the osmolality is greater than the osmolarity.

Plasma osmolality ranges from 280 to 295 mOsm/kg (not mOsm/L, as that is the unit for osmolarity!). This osmolality is consistent throughout the body compartments due to the free water-permeability of membranes separating the compartments. Plasma osmolality can be estimated from the major solutes in that compartment:

Calculated osmolality (mOsm/kg) = $2[Na^+] + [glucose] + [urea]$ (all in mmol/L)

Osmolality is regulated by osmoreceptors located outside the blood–brain barrier in the hypothalamus. These receptors are activated in the presence of an increased osmolality. This results in the release of vasopressin (antidiuretic hormone, ADH), as well as stimulation of thirst.

Smith T, Pinnock C, Lin T. *Fundamentals of Anaesthesia*, 3rd edn. Cambridge: Cambridge University Press, 2009; pp. 224–5, 510.

MTF Question 18: Non-depolarising neuromuscular blocking agents

Regarding non-depolarising neuromuscular blocking agents:

(a) The neuromuscular block is antagonised by administration of anticholinesterases
(b) Fade to a 1 Hz stimulus is present when there is partial neuromuscular block
(c) The diaphragm is paralysed at lower doses than the adductor policis muscle
(d) Post-tetanic potentiation is seen when there is partial neuromuscular block
(e) Monitoring of the adductor policis muscle is more accurate at reflecting the degree of laryngeal muscle blockade than the orbicularis oculi muscle

Answer: a,b,d

Short explanation
Neuromuscular diaphragm blockade requires two times the dose required for adductor policis muscle blockade. Facial nerve stimulation with orbicularis oculi muscle response monitoring is a better reflection of neuromuscular diaphragm and laryngeal blockade onset.

Long explanation
The use of neuromuscular blocking agents can cause problems at the end of an operation where their effects are still persisting. It is important to be aware of the means for monitoring the depth of neuromuscular blockade, which will act as a guide for timings of reversal and wakening. The administration of anticholinesterases, such as neostigmine, will reverse the neuromuscular blockade once the majority of the agent has been metabolised, by increasing the amount of available ACh to compete with the muscle relaxant. Reversal will not work, or will be incomplete, in patients who still have deep neuromuscular blockade.

A peripheral nerve stimulator should be used whenever neuromuscular blocking agents have been administered. The phase 2 block, achieved with non-depolarising agents, has certain characteristics. The basic principle is that anything which increases the amount of ACh at the neuromuscular junction, such as tetanic stimulation, will increase the observed twitch height. The two commonest nerves stimulated and their corresponding muscles observed are the facial nerve and orbicularis oculi and the ulnar nerve and adductor policis. The most important muscles to be adequately reversed are the diaphragm and intercostal muscles. The adductor policis muscle requires lower doses for paralysis than the diaphragm and so will overestimate the degree of neuromuscular blockade of the diaphragm.

The peripheral nerve stimulator can also be used at the time of administration of muscle relaxants in order to indicate whether the laryngeal muscles are adequately paralysed. For this the orbicularis oculi muscle is more accurate.

Gordon M. *Medical Pharmacology*, Chapter 20: Neuromuscular blocking drugs. Available online at www.cybermedicine2000.com/pharmacology2000/Central/NMJ/NM Jobj1.htm#Nondepolarizing Blockers (accessed 15 March 2012).
Peck T, Hill S, Williams M. *Pharmacology for Anaesthesia and Intensive Care*, 3rd edn. Cambridge: Cambridge University Press, 2008; p. 180.

MTF Question 19: Starvation

Regarding starvation:

(a) Glycogen reserves are depleted in less than 24 hours
(b) In early starvation, gluconeogenesis is the main process for glucose production
(c) Protein metabolism leads to an accumulation of acetyl-CoA and the subsequent formation of ketone bodies
(d) As starvation is prolonged, protein breakdown steadily increases
(e) An increase in plasma adrenaline levels results in an increase in plasma fatty acids

Answer: a,c,e

Short explanation

In the first 24 hours of starvation, glucose production is dependent on glycogenolysis of carbohydrate stores. If starvation lasts more than 24 hours, glucose is produced almost exclusively by gluconeogenesis. Protein metabolism decreases with prolonged starvation because of the formation of ketone bodies, primarily through fatty acid metabolism.

Long explanation

Starvation is the complete absence of dietary intake. This is different from malnutrition, where dietary intake is deficient in several dietary components.

Muscle and liver glycogen is the first energy store utilised. In early starvation, glycogenolysis exhausts the 500 g reserve of carbohydrate in less than 24 hours. During this time, only a small proportion of glucose is produced via gluconeogenesis. The next major energy source to be mobilised is free fatty acids. Mobilisation of these substrates is activated by an increase in plasma adrenaline. The free fatty acids undergo β-oxidation to produce acetyl coenzyme A (acetyl-CoA), which enters the citric acid cycle.

After approximately 24 hours of starvation, gluconeogenesis from amino acids takes over as the main process for glucose formation. This process coincides with a rise in plasma glucagon levels and a decrease in plasma insulin. Alanine is the most important amino acid for gluconeogenesis and can be formed through transamination of other amino acids. The increase in both protein and lipid metabolism leads to an excess of acetyl-CoA which overwhelms the citric acid cycle. As a result, acetyl-CoA is converted to acetoacetate and γ-hydroxybutyric acid, also known as ketone bodies. Most tissues, including the brain, can adapt to the use of ketone bodies as a source of energy.

With the high rate of ketone body formation from fatty acids, protein metabolism decreases with prolonged starvation. This corresponds to a fall in plasma glucagon levels to pre-fasting levels after approximately 10 days of fasting. This results in a decrease in gluconeogenesis as a protein-sparing mechanism.

The rate of protein metabolism is approximately 75 g/day during the first days of starvation. This decreases dramatically to 20 g/day by the third week of starvation because of the formation of ketone bodies. The 12–15 kg reserve of fatty acids, stored as adipose tissues, can produce energy for 20–25 days. During prolonged starvation, the basal metabolic rate can decrease by about 30%, mainly due to the decrease in mass of metabolically active tissues.

Power I, Kam P. *Principles of Physiology for the Anaesthetist*. London: Arnold, 2001; pp. 321–4.

MTF Question 20: EMLA and Ametop

Regarding topical anaesthetic creams for venepuncture:

(a) EMLA is a eutectic mixture, which in this context means a mixture of substances that have a lower melting point than either of the original substances

(b) Typically, EMLA causes skin blanching
(c) EMLA and Ametop should be stored in a refrigerator below 8 °C
(d) EMLA ideally requires 30 minutes to be fully effective
(e) Lidocaine 4% cream in a liposome base produces minimal skin discolouration and is effective within 30 minutes

Answer: a,b,e

Short explanation
EMLA can be stored at room temperature, but usually takes 60 minutes to be fully effective.

Long explanation
A number of proprietary products are available to aid numbing of the skin following topical application. This makes painful cutaneous procedures such as venepuncture more comfortable, and these products are particularly useful in paediatric anaesthetic practice.

EMLA is a eutectic mixture of local anaesthetics. Eutectic means a mixture of substances that display a single set of physical characteristics. In this context 2.5% lidocaine and 2.5% prilocaine in a white oil:water emulsion display a lower melting point and behave as an oil at room temperature. Individually they would appear as crystalline solids at room temperature.

Ametop is a 4% amethocaine presented as a cream. Ametop should be stored below 8 °C but EMLA can be stored at room temperature. EMLA typically causes skin blanching whilst Ametop tends to cause local erythema. Ametop is typically effective in 30–45 minutes and EMLA in 60 minutes.

LMX 4 is a new proprietary product of 4% lidocaine contained within liposomes that is now available for use in the UK. The lipid bilayers are able to enclose the water-insoluble lidocaine and improve solubility. The liposomes carry the encapsulated drug into the dermis, aiding transfer of lidocaine into the skin. Once in the skin, the liposomes also prolong the duration of action by protecting the lidocaine from metabolic degradation. LMX 4 is effective in 30 minutes, produces minimal skin blanching or erythema and can be stored at room temperature.

The MHRA assessment of LMX 4 is available online at www.mhra.gov.uk/home/groups/l-unit1/documents/websiteresources/con2033763.pdf (accessed 15 March 2012).

MTF Question 21: Medical gases

The medical gases used in anaesthetic practice include medical air, xenon and Heliox. Which of the following statements are true?

(a) Medical air is supplied to anaesthetic machines at a pressure of 7 bar
(b) Medical air is stored in cylinders with black bodies and black and white chequered shoulders at a pressure of 13 700 kPa
(c) Heliox (oxygen/helium mixture) has a lower density than oxygen and therefore is useful in conditions where flow is likely to be laminar
(d) Xenon has a low blood/gas partition coefficient and therefore offers rapid induction of anaesthesia
(e) Xenon is a more potent anaesthetic agent than nitrous oxide

Answer: d,e

Short explanation
Medical air can be supplied from cylinders with grey bodies and black and white chequered shoulders. It is supplied to the anaesthetic machine at a pressure of 4 bar.

Heliox has a lower density than oxygen and air, and therefore is useful in conditions where flow is likely to be turbulent.

Long explanation

Medical air is used frequently in combination with oxygen during anaesthesia. It is obtained from the atmosphere near to the site of compression, with care taken to avoid contamination from pollutants such as car exhaust. It is compressed to 13 700 kPa and passed through columns of alumina to remove water. It has a molecular weight of 44 kDa, a boiling point of −195 °C, a critical temperature of −149 °C and a critical pressure of 38 bar. It is stored in cylinders with grey bodies (yellow in the USA) with white and black quartered shoulders at a pressure of 13 700 kPa as a gas. It is also supplied as a piped system at a pressure of 4 bar to the anaesthetic machine and at 7 bar for surgical tools. The terminal outlets of the two supplies are different to prevent misconnection. It is used as a driving gas for ventilators, in combination with oxygen during anaesthesia and to operate power tools.

Heliox is a mixture of 21% oxygen and 79% helium. It is stored in cylinders with a black body and white and brown quartered shoulders at a pressure of 13 700 kPa as a gas. Heliox has a lower density than air and oxygen, and is therefore thought to be beneficial in conditions where turbulent flow is prominent, thus reducing the work of breathing.

Xenon is an inert, colourless, odourless gas. It has a very low blood/gas solubility of 0.14, giving it a rapid induction and elimination. It has a molecular weight of 131 Da and a boiling point of 108 °C. It is more potent than nitrous oxide, with a MAC value of 70. It is not irritant to the respiratory tract but has been shown to cause postoperative nausea and vomiting. It is non-toxic and harmless to the environment. Despite its favourable properties, xenon is not used in routine anaesthesia because of its expense and a lack of commercially available anaesthetic machines in which to use it.

Aitkenhead AR. *Textbook of Anaesthesia*, 5th edn. Edinburgh: Churchill Livingstone, 2007; p. 33.

Al-Shaikh B, Stacey S. *Essentials of Anaesthetic Equipment*, 3rd edn. Edinburgh: Churchill Livingstone, 2007; pp. 1–12.

MTF Question 22: Measurement of volume and flow in gases and liquids

Which of the following statements regarding the measurement of flow are correct?

(a) A Rotameter is a flowmeter
(b) The flutes on the bobbin or ridges on the ball of a flowmeter are required to ensure the gas passing it is turbulent in nature
(c) The Fick principle is used to calculate flow
(d) A Venturi accurately measures the flow of gas passing through it
(e) The Wright respirometer may produce inaccurate values if the flow through it is turbulent

Answer: a,c

Short explanation

At high flows, the gas in the flowmeter is turbulent by virtue of the diameter of the flowmeter at that point, not the flutes on the bobbin. The accuracy of the Venturi is dependent on the energy dissipated as heat. The Wright respirometer measures volume (not flow) and works by the migration of a vane; the flow of gas does not affect the accuracy of vane movement.

Long explanation

The flow of gases in anaesthesia can be measured using a flowmeter, a Wright peak flowmeter, a pneumotachograph, Pitot tubes or an electronic mass flowmeter. The principles of each of these measuring devices should be well understood by candidates.

The flowmeter is a variable-orifice device frequently used to measure the flow of oxygen, air and nitrous oxide delivered by the anaesthetic machine and the flow of oxygen from wall-mounted systems on the wards. A Rotameter is a flowmeter; in fact, the first is a trade name for the latter. A flowmeter usually contains a bobbin or ball. The pressure of gas beneath the bobbin or ball pushes it up the flowmeter until the force beneath it is balanced by the force of gravity pulling it back to its resting position. The variable orifice of the flowmeter means that the flow of gas past the bobbin at low flows is laminar, but at high flows it is turbulent. The flutes on the bobbin are to ensure continuous movement of the bobbin as gas passes it, showing that it is not stuck. It is the orifice of the flowmeter and not the flutes on the bobbin that is responsible for the turbulent flow.

Gas passing through a Venturi accelerates as its kinetic energy rises. This is associated with a fall in potential energy, which manifests as a fall in pressure. The fall in pressure can be used to calculate the flow, through a complex series of mathematical equations, but the accuracy varies with the degree of energy lost as heat and sound.

The Wright respirometer measures volume (not flow). Gas passing through it rotates a vane from which the measurement of volume is derived. Whether the gas is laminar or turbulent will not affect the vane rotation and therefore the measurement obtained.

The Fick principle is used to calculate blood flow either to an organ or to the body as a whole (the cardiac output). The value is calculated from the amount of a marker substance taken up by the organ in a unit of time divided by the concentration difference of that substance in the vessels to and from the organ. It is therefore a principle from which flow calculations can be made.

Davis PD, Kenny GNC. *Basic Physics and Measurement in Anaesthesia*, 5th edn. Oxford: Butterworth–Heinemann, 2003; pp. 11–35.

MTF Question 23: The gas laws

Which of the following statements regarding the gas laws are true?

(a) Boyle's law is used clinically when assessing the gas contents of an oxygen cylinder
(b) There are 6.022×10^{23} atoms of carbon in 0.012 kg of carbon-12, and this number is used in some gas calculations
(c) The third perfect gas law explains why an oxygen cylinder should not be exposed to extremes of heat
(d) A patient with a pneumothorax boards a commercial aeroplane, and suffers a cardiac arrest when the plane ascends to 32 000 feet – Charles' law explains this phenomenon
(e) At 273.15 K and 101.325 kPa, 1 mol of carbon dioxide gas will occupy 22.4 L. The same is true of 1 mol of argon gas.

Answer: a,b,c,e

Short explanation

The gas forming the pneumothorax remains at body temperature. As atmospheric pressure falls with the ascent of the aircraft, the volume of the gas in the pleural space expands, causing a tension pneumothorax, thereby obeying Boyle's law.

Long explanation

Boyle's law states that at constant temperature the volume of a given mass of gas is inversely proportional to absolute pressure. This principle is used clinically; Bourdon gauges monitor the pressure within oxygen cylinders and the correlation allows us to ascertain the volume of gas remaining within them. This is useful when trying to calculate how long an oxygen cylinder will last when delivering a given flow rate (for example, when transferring a patient out of hospital).

Boyle's law also explains why a patient with a pneumothorax at sea level will develop a tension pneumothorax at 32 000 feet. Given that body temperature, and therefore gas temperature, remains constant, the inspired air pressure falls on ascent of the plane, allowing the gas trapped between the layers of pleura to expand, forming a tension pneumothorax and resulting in a cardiac arrest. Think of what happens to your empty plastic drinks bottle as you ascend on a plane.

Charles' law states that at constant pressure the volume of a given mass of gas varies directly with absolute temperature.

The third perfect gas law states that at constant volume the absolute pressure of a given volume of gas varies directly with absolute temperature. The pressure inside an oxygen cylinder exposed to extremes of heat will increase, and therefore there is a risk of explosion.

One mole of any substance contains the same number of particles as there are atoms in 0.012 kg of carbon-12. This is Avogadro's number: 6.022×10^{23}. It is used in gas calculations when coupled with the information that 1 mol of any gas at standard temperature and pressure (273.15 K and 101.325 kPa) occupies 22.4 L.

Davis PD, Kenny GNC. *Basic Physics and Measurement in Anaesthesia*, 5th edn. Oxford: Butterworth–Heinemann, 2003; pp. 37–49.

MTF Question 24: Nitrous oxide

Which of the following statements about nitrous oxide are true?

(a) Nitrous oxide directly activates opioid receptors
(b) Nitrous oxide oxidises the cobalt ion in vitamin B_{12}
(c) Nitrous oxide should be avoided in the first trimester of pregnancy
(d) Nitrous oxide inhibits glutaminergic transmission at NMDA receptors
(e) Nitrous oxide has a direct myocardial depressant action

Answer: a,b,c,d,e

Short explanation

Nitrous oxide blocks NMDA receptors, increases endogenous opioid release and also stimulates opioid receptors directly. It inhibits DNA synthesis through the inhibition of vitamin B_{12}/methionine synthetase and is teratogenic. Its direct myocardial depressant activity is masked by an increase in sympathetic tone.

Long explanation

Nitrous oxide (N_2O) is a colourless, odourless gas which has anaesthetic and analgesic effects. Its primary site of action seems to be the NMDA glutamate receptor, where it has inhibitory properties. It also stimulates dopaminergic and α-adrenergic pathways, leading to an increase in endogenous opioid release in the midbrain, and directly activates opioid receptors in the periaqueductal grey matter. Unlike the other inhaled anaesthetic agents currently in clinical use, it does not have activity at $GABA_A$ receptors or on calcium channels at clinically relevant concentrations.

Apart from these desirable actions, N_2O also has adverse effects. It has a direct myocardial depressant action, although this is offset by the body producing an increase in sympathetic tone to produce a relatively neutral overall cardiovascular effect. Its low solubility makes it rapidly absorbed from the alveolus during induction, and the resulting concentration effect is beneficial in speeding inhalational induction; the corollary of this is the risk of diffusion hypoxia at emergence as it re-enters the alveolus equally rapidly at the end of the case. It increases the incidence of post-operative nausea and vomiting and diffuses into air-filled spaces, causing gut distension and contraindicating its use in gas-utilising ophthalmic procedures. It also oxidises the cobalt ion in vitamin B_{12}, preventing it from acting as a co-enzyme to methionine synthetase and reducing synthesis of methionine, thymidine, tetrahydrofolate and DNA. This effect is irreversible and only corrected by the production of new enzyme over several days.

Even a few hours exposure to N_2O produces megaloblastic changes in the bone marrow. Chronic exposure can produce agranulocytosis and degenerative CNS effects that resemble subacute combined degeneration of the spinal cord. Those patients who are B_{12} or folate deficient are at particular risk. Chronic occupational exposure to N_2O leads to an increased risk of miscarriage in theatre workers (no longer an issue in theatre suites with effective gas scavenging systems) and it may be teratogenic in humans so is best avoided in the first trimester of pregnancy. More holistically, N_2O is a greenhouse gas – although the overall contribution of anaesthesia to atmospheric N_2O levels is very small.

Banks A, Hardman J. Nitrous oxide. *Contin Educ Anaesth Crit Care Pain* 2005; **5**: 145–8. Available online at ceaccp.oxfordjournals.org/content/5/5/145 (accessed 15 March 2012).

Peck T, Hill S, Williams M. *Pharmacology for Anaesthesia and Intensive Care*, 3rd edn. Cambridge: Cambridge University Press, 2008.

MTF Question 25: Anticonvulsants

Regarding anticonvulsants:

(a) They act by either reducing cell membrane ion permeability, enhancing γ-aminobutyric acid receptor activity or inhibiting glutamate receptors
(b) Dosing should vary during the month in the management of catamenial epilepsy
(c) Given in pregnancy they may necessitate oral vitamin K and folic acid supplementation
(d) Carbamazepine is a first-line drug for absence seizures
(e) If a drug needs to be withdrawn rapidly because of toxicity, the patient should be immediately loaded with an alternative anticonvulsant

Answer: a,b,c,e

Short explanation
Carbamazepine is used in generalized or focal seizures but may make myoclonic or absence seizures worse.

Long explanation
Anticonvulsants act by either reducing cell membrane ion permeability (particularly sodium ions), enhancing inhibitory γ-aminobutyric acid (GABA) receptors or inhibiting excitatory neurotransmitter activity such as at glutamate receptors. The effects usually occur preferentially on cells firing at high frequency and so will target epileptic sites whilst maintaining normal physiological function.

One of the fundamental principles of anticonvulsant therapy is to try to maintain a steady level of drug. This is done through encouraging good compliance with once-a-day dosing, monotherapy and education. One of the exceptions to this is catamenial epilepsy, when seizures relate to the menstrual cycle. In this condition, dose scheduling with drugs such as clobazam will vary with the menstrual cycle through-out the month.

Choice of anticonvulsant should be tailored to the type of seizure experienced. Carbamazepine is a useful first-line drug in focal or generalised seizures but may worsen myoclonic or absence seizures.

If a patient stops taking an anticonvulsant, there is a real danger of status epilepti-cus. The only time in which it is acceptable for a patient to stop an agent immediately is in the presence of toxicity, and if this is necessary another anticonvulsant should be administered as a sensible loading dose with immediate effect.

Pregnant patients are unlikely to be taking sodium valproate because of the risk of teratogenesis. Of the other main-line anticonvulsants such as phenytoin, carbamaze-pine or barbiturates, the presence of enzyme-inducing properties correlates with low levels of serum and red blood cell folate. Additional supplements are recommended to help prevent neural tube defects. Enzyme-inducing anticonvulsants also reduce mater-nal levels of vitamin K, and the advice is usually to take oral vitamin K supplements in the last 2 weeks of pregnancy to reduce the risk of postpartum haemorrhage.

Bennett PN, Brown MJ. *Clinical Pharmacology*, 10th edn. Edinburgh: Churchill Livingstone Elsevier, 2008; pp. 372–5.

MTF Question 26: Coagulation tests

Which of the following statements are correct regarding tests of coagulation?

(a) A prolonged prothrombin time (PT) can be caused by heparin therapy
(b) A prolonged activated partial thromboplastin time (aPTT) may be due to hypofibrinogenaemia
(c) Haemophilia prolongs both PT and aPTT
(d) Thrombin time tests the conversion of prothrombin to thrombin
(e) Von Willebrand's disease affects the PT but not the aPTT

Answer: a,b

Short explanation
Thrombin time (TT) assesses the conversion of fibrinogen to fibrin. Haemophilia prolongs aPTT but does not affect PT. In von Willebrand's disease PT is unaffected, while a variable prolongation of aPTT is observed

Long explanation
Numerous tests are used to assess the function of the coagulation system. The most commonly performed tests are the prothrombin time (PT), activated partial thrombo-plastin time (aPTT) and a platelet count.

The PT is used to measure the efficiency of the extrinsic and final common pathway of coagulation. The extrinsic pathway is activated by tissue factor found extravascularly. Tissue factor acts as a cofactor for the cleavage of factor VII to VIIa, which then catalyses the activation of factor X. PT is measured by adding tissue factor to a sample of plasma. The function of thrombin (factor II), factors V, VII, X and fibrinogen is determined by PT. The speed of the extrinsic pathway is largely dependent on the activity of factor VII, which has a very short half-life. Therefore, the commonest causes of a prolonged PT include deficiencies in vitamin K (as factor VII is vitamin-K-dependent) through warfarin therapy or malabsorption. Liver failure (decreased synthesis of coagulation factors), disseminated intravascular coagulation (increased consumption) and hypofi-brinogenaemia may also result in a prolonged PT.

The aPTT is used to assess the intrinsic and final common pathway. This cascade involves the activation of factors XI, IX, VIII and X, before joining the final common pathway. A prolonged aPTT may be caused by heparin therapy, liver disease, disseminated intravascular coagulation or hypofibrinogenaemia.

Thrombin time (TT) is a less commonly performed test that assesses the conversion of fibrinogen to fibrin. A prolonged TT may be caused by hypofibrinogenaemia associated with disseminated intravascular coagulation, fibrinolytic therapy or massive transfusion. Dysfibrinogenaemia, abnormal fibrinogen, may be inherited of acquired due to liver disease, and may result in a prolonged TT.

Heparin is a naturally occurring anticoagulant that binds to and activates the inhibitory enzyme antithrombin III. The activated antithrombin III then inhibits thrombin and factors X, IX, XI and XII. As a result, exogenous heparin therapy prolongs PT, aPTT and TT.

Haemophilia can be caused by a deficiency in factor VIII (haemophilia A) or factor IX (haemophilia B). As these clotting factors are involved in the intrinsic pathway, haemophilia produces a prolonged aPTT while PT is unaffected. Von Willebrand's disease is a qualitative or quantitative deficiency in von Willebrand's factor, required for platelet adhesion. PT is unaffected, while a variable prolongation of aPTT is observed.

Smith T, Pinnock C, Lin T. *Fundamentals of Anaesthesia*, 3rd edn. Cambridge: Cambridge University Press, 2009; pp. 238–42.
Yentis S, Hirsch N, Smith G. *Anaesthesia and Intensive Care A–Z: an Encyclopaedia of Principles and Practice*, 3rd edn. Edinburgh: Butterworth–Heinemann, 2004; p. 243.

MTF Question 27: Hysteresis

Which of the following statements regarding hysteresis are true?

(a) Hysteresis of a monitoring device refers to the ability of the device to respond in both a positive and a negative direction
(b) Hysteresis is a common problem among medical monitoring devices
(c) Hysteresis in a monitoring device is a time-dependent problem
(d) The hysteresis in a system occurs because of a change in temperature
(e) Hysteresis never occurs if the value to be measured is static

Answer: e

Short explanation
Hysteresis describes the difference in the measured value when the true value is increasing compared to when it is decreasing. It is rare, and describes the accuracy of a reading at any moment in time as the system is increasing or decreasing.

Long explanation
The term *hysteresis* is familiar to most anaesthetists from their knowledge of respiratory physiology. The same term is used in the description of medical monitoring equipment, and it describes the difference in the measured value when the true value is increasing compared to when it is decreasing.

Thus, if a blood-pressure monitoring system displays no hysteresis, the true value of blood pressure is displayed as the pressure is increasing and when the pressure is decreasing. However, if hysteresis is inherent in the system, a true blood pressure of 100 mmHg may be displayed as the pressure is increasing, but when the pressure is decreasing a pressure of 110 mmHg may be displayed when the actual pressure is 100 mmHg. Thus, an accurate pressure of 100 mmHg is only displayed as the pressure is increasing.

The larger the range of pressures over which a system may operate, the greater the opportunity for hysteresis to occur. Hysteresis is therefore not a time-dependent problem; it refers to the accuracy of the system as the vector of the dependent variable is changing. It therefore requires that the value to be measured is dynamic (not static) in nature for the vector to be changing. Hysteresis is rarely a serious problem among medical devices.

Davis PD, Kenny GNC. *Basic Physics and Measurement in Anaesthesia*, 5th edn. Oxford: Butterworth–Heinemann, 2003; pp. 273–88.

MTF Question 28: Cell salvage and blood processing

Regarding the cell salvage process:

(a) Blood can be salvaged from both suction and swabs
(b) A single-lumen large-bore (4 mm) suction tube is required
(c) High vacuum suction pressures (> 150 mmHg) are required
(d) Up to one-third of the red cell mass is lost during processing
(e) A consistent quality of packed red blood cells is produced

Answer: a,d

Short explanation
A double-lumen suction tube at low vacuum pressures and a normal suction tube are both required. Several factors result in a varied quality of packed red cells for reinfusion.

Long explanation
Swabs can contain as much as 50% of total surgical blood loss. By washing the swabs and then processing the resulting wash fluid, the efficiency of the salvage can be improved significantly.

It is important to have another suction tube alongside the salvage suction tubing. This allows removal of substances that are not licensed or safe for intravenous use, such as chlorhexidine or bone cement. It is also important to remove body fluids or secretions prior to cell salvage – for example, amniotic fluid, pleural fluid or gastric secretions. These substances can be removed by normal suction tubing; however, cell salvage blood requires a specific type of tubing. It must be large-bore (> 4 mm) to minimise red cell damage, while low vacuum pressures (< 150 mmHg or 20 kPa) minimise haemolysis. This tube is double-lumen, allowing immediate mixing of an anticoagulant to the salvaged blood prior to reaching the reservoir. The anticoagulant is either citrate or heparin. In the reservoir, filtration removes large clots or debris. The filtrate passes into the separation chamber, which spins it to separate out the dense red cell mass. Most of the plasma is lost at this stage, along with up to a third of the red blood cells.

Once the maximum cell density is detected by photo-optic sensors, the washing process occurs. This removes platelets, remaining plasma, free haemoglobin, anticoagulant, fat, white cells and other waste products. The resulting packed red cells are re-suspended in normal saline ready for reinfusion to the patient. Reinfusion of salvaged blood must occur within 4 hours of processing if it is kept at room temperature. The wash volume, blood quality prior to washing, degree of concentration, surgery type and presence of contaminants all determine the quality of the salvaged blood. The haematocrit is not consistent but is usually between 0.5 and 0.7.

Lakshminarasimhan K, Wee M. Perioperative cell salvage. *Contin Educ Anaesth Crit Care Pain* 2010; **10**: 104–8. Available online at ceaccp.oxfordjournals.org/content/ 10/4/104 (accessed 15 March 2012).

MTF Question 29: Pharmacokinetic analysis

Which of the following statements regarding pharmacokinetic analysis are true?

(a) The rate constant may be expressed with units of seconds^{-1}
(b) The equation $\ln C = \ln C_0 - kt$ produces a straight line when plotted
(c) The time constant is equal to the inverse of the rate constant
(d) After one time constant, the value of the dependent variable will have fallen to approximately 37% of its initial value
(e) The rate constant represents the proportional change of the dependent variable per unit time

Answer: a,b,c,d,e

Short explanation

$\ln C = \ln C_0 - kt$ is equivalent to $y = c - mx$. Since the rate constant is the proportional change in the variable per unit time, its units are simply time^{-1}. The time constant is 1/rate constant, or $C_0 \cdot 1/e$, which equates to approximately 37% of the starting value.

Long explanation

Pharmacokinetics is the study of what happens to drugs after administration. Typically drugs go through processes of absorption, distribution, metabolism and excretion, all of which can be modelled mathematically. The underlying principle of all pharmacokinetic analysis is the exponential function; this is the mathematical function that describes the situation where the rate of change of a variable alters as the value of the variable changes. It can be written thus: $dC/dt \propto C$, where C is the variable and dC/dt is the rate of change of C.

This allows us to write the equation $dC/dt = k \cdot C$, where k is a constant (the 'rate constant' of the exponential function). This constant can be positive (implying a process where C is constantly increasing in magnitude) or negative (implying a process where C is constantly decreasing in magnitude). After intravenous administration, the plasma concentration of a drug (C) declines exponentially from its maximum value.

One can integrate the equation above to give the following equation: $C = C_0 \cdot e^{-kt}$, where C_0 is the initial concentration and $-k$ is the rate constant. This equation can be simplified by taking the natural log of each side to give: $\ln C = \ln C_0 - kt$. This equation produces a straight line since it is analogous to the equation $y = c - mx$.

One can also see that $\ln (C/C_0) = -kt$, in other words the rate constant represents the proportional change in concentration per unit time, and has the dimension of time^{-1} (i.e. units of minutes^{-1}, seconds^{-1} etc.).

The inverse of the rate constant is called the time constant (τ) and it has the dimension of time (i.e. units of minutes, seconds, etc.). τ represents the time taken for the concentration to fall to $1/e$ of its initial value (C_0). Since e is equal to approx 2.718 this means that after one τ the concentration will be approx $0.37 \cdot C_0$, or 37% of its starting value. It is also the time that it would have taken for the concentration to fall to zero if the process had continued at its initial rate of decline.

Peck T, Hill S, Williams M. *Pharmacology for Anaesthesia and Intensive Care*, 3rd edn. Cambridge: Cambridge University Press, 2008.

Roberts F, Freshwater-Turner D. Pharmacokinetics and anaesthesia. *Contin Educ Anaesth Crit Care Pain* 2007; **7**: 25–9. Available online at ceaccp.oxfordjournals.org/content/7/1/25 (accessed 15 March 2012).

MTF Question 30: Cerebrospinal fluid

Cerebrospinal fluid (CSF) provides support and protection to the central nervous system. Which of the following statements concerning CSF are true?

(a) The total volume of CSF in an adult is approximately 150 mL
(b) The pH of CSF is comparable to that of plasma
(c) The formation rate of CSF is about 1.5 mL/minute
(d) Reabsorption of CSF by the choroid plexus is a passive process
(e) CSF has an increased glucose content compared to plasma

Answer: a,b

Short explanation

CSF is produced by the choroid plexuses at a rate of 0.5 mL/minute. Reabsorption of CSF by the arachnoid villi, into the dural sinuses, is a passive process. CSF has a lower glucose concentration than plasma

Long explanation

Cerebrospinal fluid (CSF) is an ultrafiltrate that surrounds the structures of the central nervous system (CNS) and fills the cerebral ventricles. The main functions of CSF include providing protection for the CNS structures. In addition, as CSF freely communicates with CNS interstitial fluid, CSF plays a role in the control of ionic homeostasis of CNS interstitial fluid and respiratory control.

CSF is produced by the choroid plexuses in the third, fourth and lateral ventricles at a rate of 0.5 mL/minute. This results in a total production of 400–500 mL/day. The total volume of CSF in an adult is approximately 150 mL. Reabsorption of CSF by the arachnoid villi, into the dural sinuses, is a passive process. The rate of absorption increases with an increasing CSF pressure.

CSF has a similar pH to plasma, as well as a similar concentration of sodium and calcium. The osmolality of CSF is identical to that of plasma, as water freely diffuses across the blood–brain barrier. CSF has a lower concentration of glucose, potassium, chloride and lymphocytes. The protein concentration of CSF is significantly lower than that of plasma, 0.3 g/L and 70 g/L respectively. This low protein content limits the buffering capacity of the CNS interstitial fluid. Therefore, pH changes for a given $PaCO_2$ are greater in the CSF than in plasma.

Smith T, Pinnock C, Lin T. *Fundamentals of Anaesthesia*, 3rd edn. Cambridge: Cambridge University Press, 2009; pp. 230–1.

Yentis S, Hirsch N, Smith G. *Anaesthesia and Intensive Care A–Z: an Encyclopaedia of Principles and Practice*, 3rd edn. Edinburgh: Butterworth–Heinemann, 2004; p. 110.

MTF Question 31: Distribution of drugs

Which of the following statements regarding the distribution of drugs are correct?

(a) The vessel-rich body compartment comprises approximately 10% of total body mass but receives approximately 75% of the cardiac output
(b) The blood/tissue partition coefficient of a drug describes its relative distribution between body compartments at equilibrium
(c) Distribution and redistribution of drug between body compartments always uses blood as an intermediary
(d) Rate of uptake of drug into the body fat compartment is higher than into the vessel-rich compartment
(e) Drug distribution into body compartments always occurs down a concentration gradient

Answer: a,b,c

Short explanation
The body fat compartment has a lower blood supply than the vessel-rich compartment and this reduces the rate of drug entry to the tissue despite the relatively greater size of this compartment. Some drugs enter tissues by active transport mechanisms against a concentration gradient (e.g. penicillin).

Long explanation
After intravenous injection of a drug, blood levels peak rapidly and the drug is carried in the blood to tissue capillaries. The amount of blood flowing to various tissues influences how the drug enters tissues and how it is distributed between body compartments. For convenience, body compartments are often thought of as comprising a vessel-rich group (with approx 10% of total mass but 75% of blood flow) and a vessel-poor compartment largely comprising body fat. Other compartments intermediate between these extremes can also be imagined (e.g. a muscle compartment).

The high blood flow to the vessel-rich compartment causes a rapid take-up of drug into that compartment and causes the blood concentration to fall. The rate of drug transfer into the fat compartment is slower despite the greater size of this compartment because its blood flow is so poor. When the concentration in the blood falls below that in the vessel-rich tissue the flow of drug is reversed, and drug leaves the tissue to re-enter the blood. However, the blood concentration is still greater than that in the fat and other intermediate compartments, and drug continues to enter them. Eventually the drug is further redistributed from muscle and other compartments into fat, from where it is slowly returned to the blood and excreted.

The blood is always the intermediary as drug moves from one compartment to another, and certain characteristics of the drug influence the precise way that it is distributed between the body compartments.

The blood/tissue partition coefficient of the drug describes its relative distribution between body compartments at equilibrium – a low value implies a drug which readily enters tissue because of either its lipophilicity or its ability to bind to intracellular protein. Other factors influencing the movement of a drug include its molecular weight, charge and the presence of active transport mechanisms, which may be able to operate against a significant concentration gradient.

Peck T, Hill S, Williams M. *Pharmacology for Anaesthesia and Intensive Care*, 3rd edn. Cambridge: Cambridge University Press, 2008.
Smith T, Pinnock C, Lin T. *Fundamentals of Anaesthesia*, 3rd edn. Cambridge: Cambridge University Press, 2009.

MTF Question 32: Vacuum-insulated evaporator

Regarding a vacuum-insulated evaporator (VIE), which of the following statements are true?

(a) A VIE should be sited in the open air more than 6 m from any combustible material
(b) A VIE should be large enough to provide 30 days of average oxygen consumption for the site it supplies
(c) A VIE is constructed of an inner carbon steel shell and an outer stainless steel shell separated by a vacuum
(d) The pressure in a VIE is greater at the bottom of the VIE than at the top of the VIE
(e) All oxygen leaving a VIE to enter the pipeline supply of a hospital is heated

Answer: a,d,e

Short explanation

A VIE consists of an outer carbon steel shell and an inner stainless steel one separated by a vacuum, and it should be large enough to maintain a pipeline oxygen supply for 10 days of average use.

Long explanation

A vacuum-insulated evaporator (VIE) stores liquid oxygen and should contain enough to provide a pipeline oxygen supply for 10 days of average use. It should not be housed within a building and should be more than 6 m away from any combustible material. It consists of a carbon steel outer shell separated from a stainless steel inner shell by a vacuum. This vacuum prevents heat exchange between the outer and inner shells, and the space also contains perlite, a volcanic glass powder that helps to minimise heat exchange in the event of a loss of vacuum.

Oxygen leaving the VIE passes through a heater and pressure-reducing valves to ensure that the pipeline temperature and pressure of the supplied oxygen remain constant. The temperature and pressure within a VIE are –160 to –180 °C and 1050 kPa, respectively. Because of heat exchange with the atmosphere and use of the liquid oxygen there are a number of mechanisms in place to maintain this temperature and pressure. If demand is low or outside temperature is high, then the temperature of the liquid oxygen will rise and this will cause the pressure in the VIE to rise. A valve will open at pressures of approximately 1500 kPa, causing oxygen to vaporise into the atmosphere. Because of the latent heat of vaporisation involved in this process the liquid oxygen in the VIE will cool. If there is high oxygen demand or a period of cold weather, then the temperature of the liquid oxygen will fall, and this is compensated for by opening of a valve that allows liquid oxygen to leave the VIE, be vaporised and then pass back into the cylinder, thus allowing the pressure to rise again. If there is exceptional oxygen demand, then liquid oxygen can pass directly into the pipeline supply, where it is heated.

Replenishing a VIE may be problematic, as the hose between the tanker and VIE needs to be kept below the critical temperature of oxygen to maintain the oxygen in liquid form. To do this, liquid oxygen is allowed to escape from the tanker into the surrounding atmosphere, and up to 25% of the oxygen is lost in this way.

MTF Question 33: Amiodarone

Amiodarone is an acceptable first-line drug in the treatment of:

(a) Complete heart block
(b) Wolff–Parkinson–White syndrome
(c) Ventricular tachycardia
(d) Torsade de pointes
(e) Ventricular fibrillation

Answer: b,c

Short explanation

Amiodarone may induce or worsen torsades de pointes. Complete heart block is managed pharmacologically with atropine and adrenaline prior to pacing. Ventricular fibrillation is initially managed with DC shock and adrenaline.

Long explanation

Amiodarone is a class III antiarrhythmic agent that prolongs phase 3 of the cardiac action potential. The list of side effects such as skin pigmentation, corneal deposits, thyroid disturbances (both hyper- and hypo-) and pulmonary fibrosis is essential knowledge. It has increased in popularity and scope of use, despite its poor side-effect profile, because it produces minimal negative inotropy and is rarely arrhythmogenic. Amiodarone has been used for treating most tachyarrhythmias. The first-line drug for ventricular fibrillation is adrenaline with early DC cardioversion. Amiodarone is used prior to the fourth DC shock in the adult ALS algorithm. If ventricular tachycardia is pulseless, the management would be as for ventricular fibrillation. However, if the patient has good blood pressure and is in ventricular tachycardia, amiodarone is a good first-line drug treatment.

Amiodarone may be used to treat the tachycardia in patients with the ventricular pre-excitation syndrome, Wolff–Parkinson–White. The polymorphous ventricular tachycardia, torsade de pointes, may be induced or worsened by amiodarone. Initial treatment, if unstable, is DC cardioversion, and further treatment is determined by the presence or absence of a prolonged QT interval. Other tachyarrhythmias for which amiodarone is unsuitable include atrial fibrillation caused by thyrotoxicosis and the arrhythmia produced by digoxin toxicity. Drugs used in complete heart block are atropine and adrenaline until pacing is established.

Resuscitation Council Guidelines are available online at www.resus.org.uk/pages/als.pdf and www.resus.org.uk/pages/periarst.pdf (accessed 15 March 2012).

MTF Question 34: Derived SI units

Regarding derived SI units, which of the following statements are correct?

(a) 50 degrees Celsius is equivalent to 323 kelvin
(b) Both joules and electron volts are measures of energy
(c) A coulomb (C) is the quantity of electricity transported in 1 second by 1 volt
(d) A pascal (Pa) is the pressure of 1 newton per square metre
(e) A force of 1 newton (N) will give a mass of 1 kilogram an acceleration of 1 metre per second

Answer: a,b,d

Short explanation

Degrees Celsius = kelvin − 273.15. Both joules (J) and electron volts are measures of energy, with 1 electron volt being equal to 1.6×10^{-19} J. One C = 1 ampere. $1 \, Pa = 1 \, N/m^2$. $1 \, N = 1 \, kg \, m/s^2$.

Long explanation

Base SI units can be combined to derive units of measurement for other quantities. There are 22 of these derived units that have names, and a number of these (see table below) are of relevance to the anaesthetist.

The size of 1 degree Celsius (°C) is identical to the kelvin (K) and the relationship is °C = K − 273.15. A joule (J) is the energy expended when the point of application of a force of 1 newton (N) moves 1 metre (m) in the direction of the force. Both joules and electron volts are measures of energy, with one electron volt being equal to 1.6×10^{-19} J. A coulomb (C) is a measure of electrical charge or flux and therefore represents the amount of current flowing through a conductor, so it is defined in terms of amperes per second and not volts. The last option is a bit cruel, as the answer should be $kg \, m/s^2$ and not kg m/s.

Name	Symbol	Quantity	Expressed in SI base units
Hertz	Hz	Frequency	waves/s
Newton	N	Force, weight	$kg\,m/s^2$
Pascal	Pa	Pressure, stress	$kg/m/s^2$
Joule	J	Energy, work, heat	$m^2\,kg/s^2$
Watt	W	Power, radiant flux	$m^2\,kg/s^3$
Coulomb	C	Electric flux, electric charge	s A
Volt	V	Voltage, electrical potential difference, electromotive force	$m^2\,kg/s^3\,A$
Ohm	Ω	Electrical resistance, impedance, reactance	$m^2\,kg/s^3\,A^2$
Degree Celsius	°C	Temperature	K − 273.15
Tesla	T	Magnetic field strength, magnetic flux density	$kg/s^2\,A$

MTF Question 35: The analgesic ladder

The analgesic ladder:

(a) Was originally championed by the World Health Organization to give guidance for cheap effective analgesia from acute pain in the developing world
(b) Recommends the use of adjuvant therapy only once strong opioids have failed to be effective
(c) Recommends that analgesics are given only as required to avoid adverse effects
(d) Recommends the use of a maximum of only three analgesic agents at any one time
(e) Has subsequently been shown to be 80–90% effective for cancer pain

Answer: e

Short explanation
The analgesic ladder was originally designed for managing cancer pain. The ladder recommends regular analgesics rather than 'as required' prescribing, allows for more than three agents at any one time and also recommends adjuvant agents if required at any rung of the ladder

Long explanation
The analgesic ladder was first championed by the World Health Organization (WHO) in 1986 for the management of cancer pain. It has subsequently found a place as a management plan for acute pain. The plan involves the effective logical use of a few simple agents, with an escalation from drugs with low levels of adverse effects to stronger agents with correspondingly more dangerous adverse effects.

The concept involves a first rung of the ladder when a simple analgesic such as paracetamol or a non-steroidal anti-inflammatory drug (NSAID) is administered. If this is ineffective, a mild opioid such as codeine or tramadol is added in. If this remains ineffective, a stronger opioid such as morphine is added in.

The plan recommends regularly administered agents rather than drugs prescribed on an 'as required' basis. The plan does not limit the use to only one agent from each rung of the ladder, and certainly the use of paracetamol and a NSAID may be an extremely effective tactic. Adjuvant agents are included as an option on all rungs of the ladder and should be used if specifically indicated. This would include anti-depressants, anticonvulsants, steroids, muscle relaxants and non-pharmacological help such as exercise, acupuncture or psychotherapy.

In cancer patients, the WHO analgesic ladder has been found to provide effective analgesia in 80–90% of patients

WHO pain ladder. Available online at www.who.int/cancer/palliative/painladder/en/ (accessed 15 March 2012).

MTF Question 36: Amitriptyline

Common side effects of amitriptyline at therapeutic doses include:

(a) Diarrhoea
(b) Agitation
(c) Hypertension
(d) Urinary retention
(e) Blurred vision

Answer: d,e

Short explanation
Amitriptyline is a tricyclic antidepressant which typically produces a side-effect profile of muscarinic receptor blockade manifesting as urinary retention, blurred vision, constipation, sedation and postural hypotension.

Long explanation
Patients frequently present for surgery on amitriptyline. Although its use as an anti-depressant has declined since the advent of the selective serotonin reuptake inhibitors (SSRIs), it is frequently prescribed for complex or chronic pain indications. Amitriptyline is a tricyclic antidepressant which may produce a side-effect profile caused by muscarinic, histaminergic and α-adrenoreceptor blockade. Typical side effects include urinary retention, blurred vision, constipation, sedation and postural hypotension.

Agitation may be seen in patients suffering amitriptyline toxicity, along with delirium, seizures, respiratory depression and/or coma. Agitation is not commonly a feature at therapeutic doses. Cardiovascular effects of toxicity are also seen, such as sinus tachycardia, prolonged QT interval and hypertension at lower doses, progressing to ventricular arrhythmias and hypotension.

MTF Question 37: Circle system configuration

Regarding the circle system, which of the following are true?

(a) Increasing the length of the inspiratory and expiratory limbs will not alter the circuit dead space
(b) Circuit dead space will not be altered by failure of the expiratory unidirectional valve
(c) Placement of the fresh gas inlet between the patient and the expiratory unidirectional valve will allow re-breathing
(d) The adjustable pressure-limiting (APL) valve should be sited between the fresh gas inlet and the inspiratory unidirectional valve
(e) To maximise the lifespan of the CO_2 absorber, the CO_2 absorption canister should be located after the APL valve in the circle

Answer: a,c,e

Short explanation

If either of the unidirectional valves fails, re-breathing becomes possible, significantly increasing the circuit's dead space. If the APL is sited after the fresh gas flow, gas vented will include the fresh gas, reducing the efficiency of the system.

Long explanation

The essential features of a circle system are (in normal order): fresh gas inlet, breathing bag/ventilator connection, inspiratory unidirectional valve, corrugated inspiratory tubing to patient, Y-connector, corrugated expiratory tubing from patient, expiratory unidirectional valve, APL valve, and CO_2 absorber canister.

Because of the unidirectional valves, expired air can only flow into the expiratory limb, while inspired gas can only be drawn from the inspiratory limb. This limits the circuit dead space to the small area of the Y-connector. The length of the inspiratory and expiratory tubing does not therefore affect circuit dead space (but very long tubing may cause an increase in the resistance to breathing). The failure of one of the unidirectional valves may allow re-breathing, and will significantly increase circuit dead space.

If the fresh gas flow enters between the patient and the expiratory unidirectional valve, it becomes possible to inspire from the expiratory limb, resulting in re-breathing.

If the APL valve is sited after the fresh gas inlet as described, the circuit can be used safely. However, the fresh gas being delivered is vented before reaching the patient, so this is not economically the optimal conformation. For optimal efficiency, the APL valve should be located after the expiratory unidirectional valve.

By positioning the CO_2 absorber after the APL, some of the CO_2 produced by the patient will have been vented before reaching the absorber, reducing the amount that the absorber needs to take up. This results in a longer absorber lifespan.

Davey A, Diba A. Breathing systems and their components. In: *Ward's Anaesthetic Equipment*, 5th edn. Philadelphia, PA: Saunders, 2005; pp. 147–53.

MTF Question 38: Defibrillators

Regarding standard external defibrillators, which of the following are true?

(a) Direct current is used to charge the defibrillator
(b) The key component within the circuit for storing of the electrical charge is the inductor
(c) The inductor ensures that the duration of the current flow is optimum
(d) The total current produced during a shock is about 35 A
(e) The shock delivered to the patient is AC energy

Answer: c,d

Short explanation

Alternating current from the mains power supply is used to charge the capacitor within the circuit. The capacitor stores the charge before discharge. The shock delivered to the patient is DC energy.

Long explanation

Defibrillators were first used only as internal paddles, until the 1950s when the first external defibrillators became available. Initially they used alternating current, but later work demonstrated that direct current is more effective and less damaging.

The defibrillator consists of a first circuit with a power supply (usually mains AC, but battery-powered units are available) and a capacitor. Within this circuit is also a transformer (step-up), which converts mains voltage of 240 V to 5000 V. A rectifier converts this to 5000 V DC. The capacitor is charged to a potential difference of 5000–8000 V. The capacitor stores this until discharge.

The second circuit, involving the patient, contains an inductor, which ensures that the electrical pulse delivered is of optimum shape and duration. The total current produced is around 30–35 A; however, the chest wall impedance means that the amount delivered to the heart is far less. The delivered energy is important, and so the calibration of modern defibrillators is based on this. When the operator selects 360 J, this is the energy delivered to the patient. The capacitor may store more than this.

Al-Shaikh B, Stacey S. *Essentials of Anaesthetic Equipment*, 3rd edn. Edinburgh: Churchill Livingstone, 2007; pp. 205–6.
Yentis S, Hirsch N, Smith G. *Anaesthesia and Intensive Care A–Z: an Encyclopaedia of Principles and Practice*, 4th edn. Edinburgh: Churchill Livingstone, 2009; p. 161.

MTF Question 39: Hypnotics and sedatives

Which of the following statements about a sedative drug are true?

(a) Zopiclone is a benzodiazepine
(b) Plasma concentrations of zopiclone may be increased by concurrent administration of clarithromycin
(c) Zopiclone is suitable for long-term use as a night sedative
(d) Zopiclone is available as an intravenous formulation
(e) Zopiclone has active metabolites

Answer: b,e

Short explanation

Zopiclone is not structurally a benzodiazepine. Zopiclone was developed in an attempt to overcome dependence associated with benzodiazepines, but it has been found to cause dependence and is unsuitable for long-term use. It is available only as an oral formulation. Its metabolites are only weakly active at the $GABA_A$ receptor.

Long explanation

Zopiclone is not structurally a benzodiazepine but it acts via the benzodiazepine site on the $GABA_A$ receptor. It is a cyclopyrolone derivative. Zopiclone is metabolised by the CYP3A4 isoenzymes, and they are inhibited by drugs such as clarithromycin, leading to increased plasma concentrations and adverse reactions. Zopiclone was developed in an attempt to overcome dependence associated with benzodiazepines but has been found to cause dependence and is unsuitable for long-term use. Metabolites of zopiclone are weakly active at the $GABA_A$ receptor.

Futher information is available online from the US Food and Drug Administration at www.drugs.com/ppa/eszopiclone.html (accessed 15 March 2012).

MTF Question 40: Atrial fibrillation and flutter

Regarding atrial dysrhythmias:

(a) A wide QRS complex is an associated electrocardiographic feature of atrial fibrillation
(b) Atrial flutter waves are best visualised in the inferior leads
(c) Unlike atrial flutter, an isoelectric baseline is seen in atrial fibrillation
(d) The atrial rate in atrial fibrillation is typically in excess of 400 beats per minute
(e) With chronic atrial fibrillation, an enlarged left atrium would be expected on echocardiogram

Answer: b,d,e

Short explanation

Atrial fibrillation and flutter both have a baseline that is not isoelectric, and both show narrow QRS complexes (unless pre-existing or rate-related conduction abnormalities exist). The atrial rate in atrial fibrillation is typically faster than that in atrial flutter.

Long explanation

Atrial fibrillation is the most common atrial dysrhythmia, with atrial flutter the second most common. Atrial fibrillation may occur in association with chronic hypertension, pericarditis, pulmonary embolism, coronary artery disease, thyrotoxicosis and rheumatic valvular disease. The most common pathophysiologic changes include left atrial enlargement, atrial inflammation and fibrosis. On the ECG, atrial fibrillation presents with an irregularly irregular rhythm. The baseline is not isoelectric but oscillating, with fibrillatory waves of different amplitude, duration and morphology. Distinct P waves are not visible. The atrial fibrillatory rate is typically in excess of 400 beats per minute. The ventricular rate is usually slower than this due to fibrillatory impulse partially activating the AV node and making it refractory. The QRS complex is usually narrow unless there is a pre-existing or rate-related intraventricular conduction abnormality.

Atrial flutter shares many of the predisposing illnesses with atrial fibrillation. Atrial flutter is usually paroxysmal, with conversion to sinus rhythm or atrial fibrillation occurring within a few hours of onset. A regular rhythm is commonly seen in atrial flutter. As with atrial fibrillation, the baseline is not isoelectric. Atrial flutter waves (saw-tooth pattern) are best observed in the inferior leads (I, III, avF) and V_6. Symptoms are largely associated with rate, with atrial rate typically 250–350 beats per minute. Ventricular rate is usually half the atrial rate due to the physiologic 2:1 AV conduction. The QRS complex is usually narrow unless there is a pre-existing or rate-related intraventricular conduction abnormality.

Chan T, Brady W, Harrigan R, Ornato J, Rosen P. *ECG in Emergency Medicine and Acute Care*. Philadelphia, PA: Elsevier, 2005; pp. 96–101.

MTF Question 41: Hyperkalaemia

Hyperkalaemia may be secondary to:

(a) Acute kidney injury
(b) Haemolysis
(c) Alkalosis
(d) β-Blockers
(e) High-dose glucocorticoids

Answer: a,b,d

Short explanation

True hyperkalaemia may be secondary to acidosis, not alkalosis. Glucocorticoids cause movement of potassium into cells, resulting in hypokalaemia.

Long explanation

Hyperkalaemia is defined as a serum potassium > 5.0 mmol/L. The extracellular potassium accounts for less than 5% of total body potassium. True hyperkalaemia may be secondary to redistribution or impaired renal excretion. Redistribution is associated with transcellular shifts of potassium that may occur with acidosis, β-blockers and suxamethonium. Impaired renal excretion may be exogenous or endogenous (such as haemolysis or hypercatabolism) and potassium load is often a contributing factor. Impaired excretion may be due to a low aldosterone level associated with Addison's disease. Aldosterone increases the reabsorption of water and sodium with the excretion of potassium. A deficiency would therefore result in hyperkalaemia. If aldosterone levels are normal or high, impaired excretion may be secondary to primary tubular disorders, such as lupus or renal transplants, or drugs, such as spironolactone.

The careful balance of intracellular and extracellular potassium and sodium is vital to maintain the electrochemical gradients required to maintain the resting membrane potential of a cell. As extracellular potassium increases, the resting membrane potential becomes less negative. This change can disrupt cell excitability, leading to a delay in action potential propagation and prolonged depolarisation. Clinical effects may include muscle weakness and paralysis. Myocardial depression associated with hyperkalaemia is illustrated by changes in the ECG: peaked T waves, absent P waves, widened QRS complexes and conduction abnormalities may be seen.

β-Adrenergic agonists, such as salbutamol, and glucocorticoids cause movement of potassium into cells, resulting in hypokalaemia.

Banerjee A. *Clinical Physiology: an Examination Primer*. Cambridge: Cambridge University Press, 2005.

Parham W A, Mehdirad A A, Biermann K M, Fredman C S. Hyperkalemia revisited. *Tex Heart Inst J* 2006; **33**: 40–7.

MTF Question 42: Capnography

Regarding capnography, which of the following are true?

(a) An upward slope in phase 3 may indicate uneven emptying of alveoli
(b) A difference of > 0.7 kPa between arterial carbon dioxide and end-tidal carbon dioxide is normal
(c) End-tidal carbon dioxide is always lower than alveolar carbon dioxide
(d) It is often inaccurate in neonates
(e) V/Q mismatch would decrease the difference between alveolar and end-tidal carbon dioxide

Answer: a,c,d

Short explanation

Alveolar carbon dioxide is diluted with dead-space gas from conducting airways and is higher than end-tidal; however, the difference should be 0.4–0.7 kPa. This difference is increased in V/Q mismatch. In paediatrics, carbon dioxide is diluted by fresh gas flow, causing an inaccurate result.

Long explanation

Capnography is the measurement and pictorial display of carbon dioxide concentration. It appears as a square waveform with four phases. Phase 1 is the baseline, which occurs during inspiration. This baseline will be raised if re-breathing of carbon dioxide occurs. Phase 2 is the exhalation of dead-space gas, which will contain no carbon dioxide. Phase 3 is the exhalation of alveolar gas. This is the plateau phase. If alveoli do not empty evenly or if there is obstruction to exhalation, there will be sloping of this phase. Phase 4 is the fall back to baseline for the onset of inspiration.

Alveolar carbon dioxide is diluted with dead-space gas from conducting airways and is therefore always higher than end-tidal carbon dioxide; however, the difference should only be 0.4–0.7 kPa. This difference is increased in V/Q mismatch.

In paediatrics, higher respiratory rates and lower tidal volumes result in carbon dioxide levels being diluted by fresh gas flow and hence an inaccurate result. Accuracy can be improved by the use of special adapters in neonates to reduce the dead space and to allow the capnograph to be attached closer to the trachea.

Al-Shaikh B, Stacey S. *Essentials of Anaesthetic Equipment*, 2nd edn. Edinburgh: Churchill Livingstone, 2002; pp. 117–20.
Yentis S, Hirsch N, Smith G. *Anaesthesia and Intensive Care A–Z: an Encyclopedia of Principles and Practice*, 3rd edn. Edinburgh: Butterworth–Heinemann, 2004; pp. 85, 87.

MTF Question 43: Measurement of pH

Regarding the measurement of pH, which of the following are true?

(a) pH is measured by the Severinghaus electrode
(b) pH is the logarithm to base 10 of hydrogen ion concentration measured in nmol/L
(c) Older samples will have a higher pH
(d) An arterial blood gas analyser will measure pH and base excess
(e) An increase in temperature will increase dissociation of acids

Answer: e

Short explanation

The Severinghaus electrode is used to measure carbon dioxide tension. The pH is the negative logarithm to base 10 of hydrogen ion concentration. Older samples will have a lower pH as metabolism in cells continues. Base excess is not measured but is a derived value.

Long explanation

The Severinghaus electrode is a modified pH electrode. It consists of a pH-sensitive glass electrode, separated from the sample by a carbon-dioxide-permeable membrane. It is used to measure the carbon dioxide tension of a sample.

The pH is the negative logarithm to base 10 of hydrogen ion concentration measured in nanomoles per litre. As the hydrogen ion concentration increases, the pH decreases. A pH of 7.4 is equal to a hydrogen ion concentration of 40 nmol/L.

Older blood samples will continue to metabolise, using oxygen and producing carbon dioxide. For this reason older samples will have a lower oxygen content and a higher carbon dioxide content and hence a lower pH. Samples should be stored on ice if a delay in processing is expected. It should also be noted that the presence of air bubbles in a blood sample would falsely increase the oxygen tension and lower the carbon dioxide tension. Care should be taken to expel air from samples.

Arterial blood gas analysers measure pH, partial pressures of oxygen and partial pressures of carbon dioxide. Bicarbonate, standard bicarbonate, base excess and oxygen saturations are all derived values. Increases in temperature will increase the dissociation of acids. pH electrodes are maintained at 37 °C for this reason. Values may also need to be corrected if the patient is hypothermic or hyperthermic.

Al-Shaikh B, Stacey S. *Essentials of Anaesthetic Equipment*, 2nd edn. Edinburgh: Churchill Livingstone, 2002; pp. 164–7.
Davies PD, Kenny GNC. *Basic Physics and Measurement in Anaesthesia*, 5th edn. London: Butterworth–Heinemann, 2003; pp. 211–13.

MTF Question 44: Thyroid hormones – calcitonin

Calcitonin:

(a) Plays a major role in calcium homeostasis
(b) Is secreted by C cells
(c) Is secreted by the thyroid gland, lung and intestinal tract
(d) Is secreted by parafollicular cells
(e) Increases blood levels of calcium by activation of osteoclasts

Answer: b,c,d

Short explanation
Calcitonin plays only a minor role in calcium homeostasis. The effects of calcitonin include reducing plasma calcium levels through inhibition of osteoclasts.

Long explanation
In addition to thyroxine the thyroid also produces calcitonin. Calcitonin is secreted by the C cells, which are also known as the parafollicular cells. The C cells are located between thyroid follicles.

Calcitonin is a 32 amino acid peptide which is cleaved from a larger prohormone. The single disulphide bond causes the amino terminus to assume the shape of a ring. The calcitonin receptor is a seven-transmembrane G-protein-coupled receptor. Calcitonin is not a major contributor to calcium homeostasis in the body. It does reduce plasma calcium levels via effects on two main organs. Calcitonin inhibits the action of osteoclasts and therefore reduces bone resorption and calcium release from bones. Calcitonin also acts on the kidney and inhibits tubular resorption of calcium and phosphorus, leading to increased rates of loss of these ions in the urine.

Calcitonin is released from the thyroid gland and also the lungs and gastrointestinal tract. The extracellular concentration of ionised calcium is the most important factor controlling calcitonin release. Calcitonin can be used therapeutically in patients with hypercalcaemia.

Bowen R. Calcitonin. Available online at www.vivo.colostate.edu/hbooks/pathphys/ endocrine/thyroid/calcitonin.html (accessed 15 March 2012).

MTF Question 45: Simple mechanics – mass

Which of the following statements regarding mass are correct?

(a) Mass varies under conditions of differing gravity
(b) The SI unit for mass is the gram
(c) The unit for mass is based on a prototype held at Sèvres near Paris
(d) The term weight can be used interchangeably with the term mass
(e) Mass can be described as the gravitational force acting on an object

Answer: c

Short explanation

Mass is a constant and does not vary with gravity. The SI unit is the kilogram. The term weight is often mistakenly used interchangeably with the term mass but this is incorrect. Weight is the gravitational force acting on an object.

Long explanation

Mass is the property of an object that remains constant no matter where the object is situated. It can be defined as the amount of matter contained in a body and has the dimensions [M]. The SI unit of mass is the kilogram; this is indeed based on the mass of a 1 kg prototype held at Sèvres near Paris. The gram is 1/1000 of a kilogram.

Mass and weight are often used interchangeably in everyday language, but this is incorrect. Weight is the gravitational force acting on an object and can be described as the mass multiplied by the acceleration due to gravity. The weight of a body of mass 1 kg is 1 kg weight (kilogram force). Therefore this suggests that weight varies with varying gravity; hence the reason that your weight would be less on the moon than on earth.

Masses of gases are described in a different way, as it is more convenient to use a concept related to the number of molecules, i.e. the mole. A mole is the quantity of a substance containing the same number of particles as there are atoms in 0.012 kg (12 g) of carbon-12.

Smith T, Pinnock C, Lin T. *Fundamentals of Anaesthesia*, 3rd edn. Cambridge: Cambridge University Press, 2009; p. 731.

Yentis S, Hirsch N, Smith G. *Anaesthesia and Intensive Care A–Z: an Encyclopaedia of Principles and Practice*, 3rd edn. Edinburgh: Butterworth–Heinemann, 2004; p. 547.

MTF Question 46: Glyceryl trinitrate

Glyceryl trinitrate:

(a) Is a pro-drug
(b) If administered as a patch, should be removed before defibrillation to avoid risk of explosion
(c) Principally exerts its antianginal effect by dilating the venous side of the circulation
(d) As an intravenous infusion may be limited in duration by the risk of developing methaemoglobinaemia
(e) Is contraindicated if the patient is found to have a failing left ventricle

Answer: a,c,d

Short explanation

Any patch containing metal should be removed prior to defibrillation because of the risk of burns, but a glyceryl trinitrate patch will not explode. Glyceryl trinitrate is indicated rather than contraindicated for patients developing left ventricular failure.

Long explanation

Glyceryl trinitrate (GTN) is a potent, short-acting vasodilator that is indicated for angina and left ventricular failure. Glyceryl trinitrate is a pro-drug. Pro-drugs are inactive or significantly less active in their administered form and require some form of chemical change, usually metabolism, to form the active drug. Glyceryl trinitrate as a molecule is relatively inactive and requires denitration to produce nitric oxide, the chemical which causes vasodilation.

The urban myth about exploding defibrillated GTN patches is not true. It was investigated on the television program *Mythbusters* and found to be impossible. However, any patch containing metal should be removed prior to defibrillation because of the risk of burns.

Although glyceryl trinitrate does work in angina as a coronary arterial dilator, its principal mechanism is by causing venodilation, reducing venous return, and therefore reducing left ventricular work. Long-term intravenous infusion of glyceryl trinitrate has been discouraged because of the risk of methaemoglobinaemia.

MTF Question 47: Raised intracranial pressure

Normal intracranial pressure (ICP) ranges from 5 to 15 mmHg. Regarding raised ICP, which of the following statements are correct?

(a) Headache associated with raised ICP is classically worse in the morning and relieved by stooping forward
(b) Cushing's reflex consists of marked hypertension and tachycardia
(c) Benign intracranial hypertension can lead to permanent blindness and is most common amongst young women
(d) Management of a patient with raised ICP includes encouragement of venous drainage by keeping patients slightly head-down
(e) Raised ICP may be a feature of Dandy–Walker syndrome

Answer: c,e

Short explanation
The headache associated with raised ICP is classically worse in the morning and on stooping and straining. Cushing's reflex consists of hypertension and bradycardia. Management of raised ICP employs a head-up position to encourage venous drainage.

Long explanation
Intracranial pressure (ICP) is the pressure inside the cranial vault relative to atmospheric pressure. The normal range is 5–10 mmHg. Clinical features of raised ICP include headache, nausea and vomiting and confusion. The headache described is classically worse in the morning and on straining or stooping. Signs of raised ICP include papilloedema, impaired consciousness and hypertension and bradycardia (Cushing's reflex). Papilloedema describes swelling of the optic discs seen with an ophthalmoscope and may take 24 hours of raised ICP to develop. Cushing's reflex was first described by Harvey Cushing, an American neurosurgeon, in 1902, and it describes a clinical syndrome of hypertension and bradycardia associated with an acutely raised ICP. It is thought to be due to the effect of local hypoxia and hypercapnia on the vasomotor centre as the cerebral perfusion pressure falls. During the later stages of raised ICP hypotension, coma, irregular respiration or apnoea and fixed, dilated pupils may develop.

The intracranial contents can be divided into four compartments: solid material, tissue water, cerebrospinal fluid (CSF) and blood. Raised ICP can be caused by an increase in volume of any of these intracranial compartments without a compensatory decrease in another compartment.

Increased blood volume may be caused by increased cerebral blood flow or impaired venous drainage, for example during coughing, straining, with kinked jugular veins and in the head-down position. Increased volume of brain tissue could be caused by tumour, abscess or haematoma formation, or by cerebral oedema.

Causes of increased CSF volume can be divided into congenital and acquired. Congenital causes include Dandy–Walker syndrome (obstruction of fourth ventricle outlet), Arnold–Chiari syndrome (herniation of cerebellar tonsils through the foramen magnum) or by a narrow aqueduct. Acquired causes include meningitis with adhesions, surgery, head injury, subarachnoid haemorrhage and tumour.

Benign intracranial hypertension is associated with none of the causes mentioned above and is most common in young women. It can cause permanent visual impairment due to optic nerve damage. Its management includes repeated lumbar-puncture CSF drainage, corticosteroids and shunt insertion.

Smith T, Pinnock C, Lin T. *Fundamentals of Anaesthesia*, 3rd edn. Cambridge: Cambridge University Press, 2009; pp. 403–4.

Yentis S, Hirsch N, Smith G. *Anaesthesia and Intensive Care A–Z: an Encyclopaedia of Principles and Practice*, 3rd edn. Edinburgh: Butterworth–Heinemann, 2004; pp. 281–2.

MTF Question 48: Henderson–Hasselbalch equation

Regarding the Henderson–Hasselbalch equation:

(a) Provided the ratio of HCO_3^-/CO_2 remains constant, the pH of a system also remains constant
(b) The equation can be used to calculate the amount of acid or base required to make a solution a specific pH
(c) For a weak acid, if the pH is less than the pKa, molecules are more ionised
(d) The Henderson–Hasselbalch equation is based on the dissociation equation of carbonic acid
(e) The Henderson–Hasselbalch equation demonstrates why local anaesthetics are less ionised with increasing acidity

Answer: a,b,d

Short explanation

The Henderson–Hasselbalch equation describes the relationship between dissociated and undissociated acid or base. For a weak acid, if the pH is less than the pKa, the solution is more un-ionised. The opposite is true for weak bases (including most local anaesthetics).

Long explanation

The Henderson–Hasselbalch equation describes the relationship between dissociated and undissociated acid or base:

$$pH = pKa + \log \{[\text{proton acceptor}]/[\text{proton donor}]\}$$

where the pKa is the pH at which 50% of molecules are ionized.

The equation was originally described in relation to any buffer system but now often specifically applies to the bicarbonate buffer system. It is therefore based on the dissociation equation of carbonic acid:

$$CO_2 + H_2O \leftrightarrow H^+ + HCO_3^-$$

Rearranging this equation and taking the logarithms on both sides gives you the Henderson–Hasselbalch equation

$$pH = pKa + \log \{[HCO_3^-]/[H_2CO_3]\}$$

In accordance with this equation, the pH of a system will stay constant provided the ratio of HCO_3^-/CO_2 also remains constant. This is the principle behind compensation for metabolic disturbances in the body. This equation can also be applied to calculate the amount of acid or base required to make a buffer solution a specific pH. For a weak acid, if the pH is less than the pKa, the solution is more un-ionised, while the solution is more ionised if the pH is greater than the pKa. The opposite is true for weak bases such as most local anaesthetics (pKa 7.6–8.9). This explains why local anaesthetics are more ionised with a lower pH, and therefore less effective in acidic, infected tissue, as the large fraction of ionised molecules cannot passively move intracellularly where they block sodium channels.

Yentis S, Hirsch N, Smith G. *Anaesthesia and Intensive Care A–Z: an Encyclopaedia of Principles and Practice*, 3rd edn. Edinburgh: Butterworth – Heinemann, 2004.

MTF Question 49: Pipeline and suction systems

Regarding pipelines and medical suction, which of the following are true?

(a) All piped gases are supplied to theatre at 4 kPa
(b) The gas outlet at the wall consists of non-interchangeable screw-thread (NIST) connections specific for each gas
(c) The gas outlet at the wall consists of Schrader sockets specific for each gas
(d) Piped suction systems must have a minimum flow rate of 35 L/min
(e) Piped suction systems must generate a minimum of 7 kPa of negative pressure

Answer: c,d

Short explanation
Air is supplied at 4 kPa, and also at 7 kPa for surgical instruments. All other gases are supplied at 4 kPa. The wall connections are Schrader sockets that are specific to each gas, while the NIST connectors connect the hose to the anaesthetic machine. Medical suction via the piped system must generate a negative pressure of 80 kPa and a flow rate of 35 L/min.

Long explanation
The piped medical gas and vacuum (PMGV) supplies air at both 4 kPa and 7 kPa (for surgical instruments). All other gases are supplied at 4 kPa.

Anaesthetists are responsible for gases supplied from the wall outlet to the anaesthetic machine; prior to the wall, pharmacy and medical engineering take responsibility for the safety of piped gases. The wall outlet consists of a Schrader socket that has an index collar specific for each gas. The probes for the sockets are individual to each gas, so hoses cannot be connected to the wrong outlet. Connections at the anaesthetic machine are permanently fixed and are also specific to each gas; the non-interchangeable screw-thread (NIST) connection ensures this.

The hoses for gases are colour-coded: oxygen is white, air is black and white, nitrous oxide is French blue, Entonox is French blue and white. It medical vacuum is yellow.

Piped suction is available in all hospitals. It consists of a central reservoir with a high-displacement pump that must be able to generate a negative pressure of 80 kPa and a flow rate of 35 L/min.

Al Shaikh B, Stacey S. *Essentials of Anaesthetic Equipment*, 3rd edn. Edinburgh: Churchill Livingstone, 2007; pp. 6–7.

MTF Question 50: Omeprazole

Omeprazole:

(a) Activates the H^+/K^+-ATPase in parietal cells
(b) Is degraded by a low pH

(c) Leads to elevated gastrin levels
(d) As a sole agent for the treatment of duodenal ulcers heals the majority of patients within 4 weeks
(e) Is not used prior to caesarean section because of the risk of fetal bradycardia

Answer: b,c,d

Short explanation
Omeprazole inhibits the H^+/K^+-ATPase in parietal cells and has not been adopted in obstetric practice because it is slightly less effective than H_2 antagonists.

Long explanation
Omeprazole was the first commercially available proton pump inhibitor (PPI). A number of other PPIs are now available. All the other PPIs have the same efficacy and similar adverse-effect profiles.

Indications for the use of omeprazole include for the treatment of duodenal or gastric ulcers, for gastro-oesophageal reflux disease, erosive oesophagitis or pathological hypersecretory conditions such as Zollinger–Ellison syndrome. In the treatment of duodenal ulcers, omeprazole heals the majority of ulcers within 4 weeks, with a small group requiring a further 4-week course of tablets. In cases caused by *Helicobacter pylori*, combination therapy with clarithromycin reduces recurrence, and triple therapy with the further addition of amoxycillin reduces the risk of clarithromycin resistance.

Omeprazole works by irreversibly inactivating the H^+/K^+-ATPase in parietal cells. The pure drug is degraded at low pH and so is administered as an enteric coated tablet. As omeprazole's main effect is to raise gastric pH, as time passes, and pH rises, less drug is deactivated, so increasing the drug's bioavailability. Omeprazole is absorbed from the gastrointestinal tract once it has passed through the stomach and then enters the systemic circulation. It then diffuses into the parietal cells, where it is concentrated. Gastrin is secreted in response to rising gastric pH. Raised gastrin has been postulated as a possible mechanism by which PPIs might cause mailgnancy as gastrin promotes growth of gastric epithelium.

Omeprazole has never really caught on in obstetric anaesthesia. It has not been demonstrated to be harmful to the fetus, but the body of research evidence is very small. It was found in one study to be not as effective as the H_2 antagonists in raising gastric pH before caesarean section, and, in keeping with a lot of obstetric pharmacology, has not been adopted over the tried and tested agents as it does not confer a substantial advantage.

Bennett PN, Brown MJ. *Clinical Pharmacology*. 10th edn. Edinburgh: Churchill Livingstone Elsevier, 2008; pp. 563–4.
FDA advice available online at www.drugs.com/pro/omeprazole.html (accessed 15 March 2012).

MTF Question 51: Pre- and post-renal kidney injury

Regarding acute kidney injury:

(a) A high urinary osmolality and sodium concentration would be expected in pre-renal injury
(b) The most common causes are pre-renal in origin
(c) Anuria is often observed in acute tubular necrosis
(d) In post-renal injury, a normal plasma creatinine suggests mild disease with minimal change in the glomerular filtration rate
(e) Pre-renal injury is associated with both conditions of volume depletion and overload

Answer: b,d,e

Short explanation
Pre-renal injury is observed in the setting of absolute volume depletion. It is charac-
terised by a high urine osmolality and a urine sodium concentration < 20 mmol/L.
Anuria is usually suggestive of post-renal obstruction. In acute tubular necrosis, a form
of intrinsic renal failure, the urine volume may be normal or patients may be oliguric.

Long explanation
Acute kidney injury (AKI) is a rapid onset of deterioration in renal function. It is largely
classified as pre-renal (disruption in renal blood flow), intrinsic (renal) and post-renal
(obstruction of urine flow).

Pre-renal kidney injury represents the most common causes of AKI. It may develop
in the setting of volume depletion (e.g. haemorrhage, gastrointestinal loss, renal loss,
cutaneous loss), decreased cardiac output (e.g. myocardial infarction, congestive heart
failure, pulmonary embolus), systemic vasodilation (sepsis, anaphylaxis, anaesthesia),
afferent or efferent renal arteriolar vasoconstriction (drugs) or renal artery obstruction.
If the condition is not treated, it will lead to intrinsic injury.

Post-renal injury results from a mechanical obstruction to the urinary collecting
system and outflow tract. This includes the renal pelvis, ureters, bladder and urethra. If
the obstruction is unilateral, a rise in serum creatinine may not be observed despite a
significant reduction in glomerular filtration rate.

It is important to establish the diagnosis of renal function deterioration, as both pre-
and post-renal causes are potentially reversible before renal failure has become established. Diagnosis may be aided by the clinical history, including urine output.
Examination of the urine sediment may identify casts associated with a particular
disease process.

Plasma and urine indices can help differentiate between pre-renal and renal processes. Due to the decreased blood flow associated with pre-renal injury, there is a
related decrease in the glomerular filtration rate. This acts as a stimulus for salt and
water retention. As a result, urine osmolality exceeds 500 mOsm/kg (greater than
plasma osmolality) and urine sodium concentration is less than 20 mmol/L. Anuria
is usually suggestive of post-renal obstruction. In acute tubular necrosis, a form of
intrinsic renal failure, the urine volume may be normal or patients may be oliguric.

Andreoli T, Carpenter C, Griggs R, Loscalzo J. *Cecil Essentials of Medicine*, 5th edn.
Philadelphia, PA: Saunders, 2001; pp. 283–8.

MTF Question 52: Sevoflurane

Which of the following statements about sevoflurane are true?

(a) Sevoflurane increases respiratory dead space
(b) Sevoflurane produces carbon monoxide when combined with dry sodalime
(c) Compound A production limits the use of sevoflurane in humans
(d) Sevoflurane is not suitable for use in head-injured patients since it raises the
intracranial pressure
(e) Sevoflurane has a saturated vapour pressure of 20.9 kPa and a blood/gas partition
coefficient of 0.69

Answer: a,b,e

Short explanation
Sevoflurane (saturated vapour pressure 20.9 kPa) is a bronchodilator, and hence it
increases dead space. Carbon monoxide production is enhanced by dry conditions, high

temperatures and the presence of sodium or potassium hydroxide. Compound A is not produced in levels toxic to humans. It does not raise the intracranial pressure significantly below 1 MAC.

Long explanation

Sevoflurane is a halogenated ether with a saturated vapour pressure of 20.9 kPa and a blood/gas partition coefficient (BGPC) of 0.69. It has an onset of action faster than isoflurane (BGPC 1.43) but not as rapid as desflurane (BGPC 0.42). Its MAC is 2.0%, indicating lower potency than isoflurane. It does not produce epileptogenic EEG activity or have any analgesic effects. It raises cerebral blood flow and intracranial pressure but this effect is minimal below 1 MAC. It causes little cardiovascular instability compared to isoflurane and desflurane, lowering the systemic vascular resistance through vasodilation while leaving the cardiac output unchanged. It does not cause coronary vasodilation and coronary blood flow is unaffected, while the heart rate is reduced (lowering myocardial oxygen demand and enhancing myocardial oxygenation).

Sevoflurane reduces tidal volume and respiratory rate and relaxes bronchial smooth muscle, increasing respiratory dead space. It attenuates the respiratory response to hypercarbia and hypoxia. It relaxes uterine smooth muscle in a similar manner to other inhaled agents, increasing the risk of bleeding after obstetric procedures, and potentiates neuromuscular blockade through inhibition of calcium channels. In common with the other volatile agents it is a trigger for malignant hyperpyrexia in susceptible individuals. It has a higher degree of hepatic metabolism (around 3%) than any other agent except halothane, producing hexafluoroisopropanol (which is potentially hepatotoxic but rapidly conjugated in the liver) and inorganic fluoride ions. With prolonged sevoflurane anaesthesia (>7 MAC hours) the plasma fluoride concentration can approach levels (>40 µg/L) causing a reversible nephropathy and ADH-resistant polyuria.

Sevoflurane becomes degraded by contact with carbon dioxide absorbers in anaesthetic circle systems to form several potentially toxic products (compounds A–E). Compound A is produced most readily and causes nephrotoxicity in rats; however, it does not reach toxic levels in humans during clinical applications and no evidence of human nephrotoxicity has been demonstrated. Carbon monoxide can also be produced by contact with carbon dioxide absorbers, although the levels rarely seem to reach significance. Dry absorber material, high temperatures and the presence of sodium and potassium hydroxide all increase the rate of carbon monoxide production.

Moppett I. Inhalational anaesthetics. *Anaesth Intens Care Med* 2008; **9**: 567–72.
Smith T, Pinnock C, Lin T. *Fundamentals of Anaesthesia*, 3rd edn. Cambridge: Cambridge University Press, 2009.

MTF Question 53: Safety features of flowmeters

Regarding safety features of the flowmeter bank on an anaesthetic machine, which of the following are true?

(a) Pressing the control valve spindle in will not alter gas flow rates
(b) Flowmeters can be interchanged to allow measurement of different gases
(c) The oxygen flow control knob must be octagonal in profile
(d) Oxygen flows into the back-bar manifold before (upstream of) any other gases
(e) The internal surface of the flowmeter tube is sometimes coated with gold

Answer: c,e

Short explanation

Standards allow up to 10% flow change if pressure is applied to the control knob. The flowmeter calibration is gas-specific, and they are non-interchangeable. Oxygen flows into the manifold last. There may be a thin (invisible) gold coating inside the flowmeter tube to prevent build-up of static electricity.

Long explanation

Flow control valves in the UK have to meet the standards BS 4272 and EN ISO 606601-2-13. One of the requirements is that when axial push or pull forces are applied to the control knob, the maximum variation in flow will not be greater than 10%. Another is that the oxygen flow control knob differs from the others to make it easily locatable. It must have an octagonal profile, must stand out from the other knobs by at least 2 mm, and must have a larger diameter than the other knobs.

The Rotameter is a constant-pressure, variable-orifice, flowmeter. For the pressure to remain constant across a range of orifices and flows, it must be calibrated to a gas with known viscosity and density. Changing the gas will therefore produce an inaccurate result. Misconnection is normally impossible, with glass sight tubes of different diameters or pin-index systems.

In the UK, the oxygen flowmeter is on the left. If a leak were to develop in another flowmeter, oxygen would be lost first, potentially leading to a hypoxic mixture. To avoid this problem, internal baffles are sited above the flowmeter block, so that oxygen is delivered last, downstream of the other gases. Because the bobbin is constantly rotating, static electricity can build up. This can cause significant inaccuracy (up to 35%). Several techniques of dissipating static build-up exist, including wires at the top and bottom of the tube, or an invisibly thin coating of gold on the inside.

Davey A, Diba A. *Ward's Anaesthetic Equipment*, 5th edn. Philadelphia, PA: Saunders, 2005; pp. 58–9, 104–7.

MTF Question 54: Basic principles of electricity and magnetism

Which of the following statements correctly describe the principles of magnetism?

(a) A conductor of electricity can create a magnetic field without an external power source
(b) A magnet can create an electric current in a conductor without an external power source
(c) The unit of magnetic flux is the tesla
(d) The strength of the induced magnetic field in the galvanometer increases as the current through the wire increases
(e) The flow of blood generates an electric current when placed parallel to a magnetic field

Answer: b,d

Short explanation

An electric conductor will produce a magnetic field when current flows through it. A changing magnetic field will induce a current in a conductor surrounding it. The unit of magnetic flux is the weber; flux density is measured in tesla. The flow of blood may generate an electric current when placed perpendicular to a magnetic field.

Long explanation

A conductor can generate a magnetic field when an electric current is passed through it; so if a current is passed through a wire, a magnetic field is generated. This magnetic field may be focused into a manageable entity by winding the wire into a coil.

The magnetic field created on passing a current through the wire is greatest within the core of the coil. A magnet would theoretically create an electric current in a conductor if a magnet moves within the conductor. So if a magnet moves within a coil of wire, the changing magnetic field induces an electric current within the wire. This is the way old-fashioned bike lights worked. As the bike wheel rotated, a magnet in contact with the wheel spun. The magnet was surrounded by coils of wire and the process of rotation of the magnet within the coils induced an electric current within the coils, which was then used to power a light.

The magnetic field strength is the strength of the field within a vacuum. The magnetic flux is the strength of the field in any material. The unit of magnetic flux is the weber (Wb), 1 Wb being that flux that induces an electromotive force of 1 volt in a single turn of wire, as the flux decreases uniformly to zero in 1 second. The tesla is the unit of magnetic flux density, i.e. Wb/m^2.

The principles of magnetism are used in the galvanometer and the electromagnetic flowmeter. In the galvanometer, a coil of wire is placed in a magnetic field. As electric current flows through the coil, the induced magnetic field that results interacts with the fixed field of the permanent magnet to produce a force which causes the coil of wire to rotate. The amount of rotation is proportional to the current in the wire, the induced magnetic field and in turn the rotation of the coil and needle, and thus the device is used as a measure of current. The magnet surrounding the coil has a fixed magnetic flux. The electromagnetic flowmeter relies on the principle that blood is a good conductor of electricity. When a vessel is placed perpendicular to the flow of blood, a potential difference may be recorded across the vessel, the size of which is proportional to the average speed of blood flow within the vessel.

Davis PD, Kenny GNC. *Basic Physics and Measurement in Anaesthesia*, 5th edn. Oxford: Butterworth–Heinemann, 2003; pp. 149–64.

MTF Question 55: Heat conduction

Regarding conduction, which of the following statements are correct?

(a) Conduction is the most important route for heat loss during anaesthesia
(b) Gases are poor conductors of heat
(c) Heat loss via conduction is reduced by warming blankets
(d) Children and the elderly are at increased risk of hypothermia during anaesthesia
(e) Warming irrigating fluids reduces heat losses by conduction

Answer: b,d,e

Short explanation
Conduction is not an important route for heat loss from the body. Heat loss via radiation is reduced by the use of warming blankets.

Long explanation
There are four main routes for heat loss from the body under anaesthesia: radiation, convection, evaporation of water and heat loss through respiration. Conduction is not an important route per se and is thought to account for about 3% of the heat loss experienced. Conduction occurs when heat energy is transferred from one solid body to another, whereby there is transfer of the energy of motion of molecules to adjacent molecules. Metals are particularly good conductors of heat, whereas gases are poor conductors and act as insulators.

The amount of heat transferred by conduction is related to the area of the body exposed to a cooler solid object, and therefore reducing this contact will reduce the heat lost via this route. Heat loss via conduction is increased by the use of cool irrigating fluids.

Heat loss in theatre may lead to hypothermia if excessive for many reasons. It is therefore imperative to recognise those patients at particularly high risk, including children and the elderly, severely ill patients with malnutrition, those undergoing prolonged surgery and those with large volumes of blood loss. Steps should be taken to measure the temperature under anaesthesia, and care should be taken to avoid excessive heat loss and encourage warming.

Davis PD, Kenny GNC. *Basic Physics and Measurement in Anaesthesia*, 5th edn. Oxford: Butterworth–Heinemann, 2003; pp. 103–4.
Yentis S, Hirsch N, Smith G. *Anaesthesia and Intensive Care A–Z: an Encyclopaedia of Principles and Practice*, 3rd edn. Edinburgh: Butterworth–Heinemann, 2004; p. 242.

MTF Question 56: Measuring functional residual capacity

Which of the following statements are correct regarding the measurement of functional residual capacity (FRC)?

(a) Helium is used for the gas dilution technique because of its low solubility in blood
(b) Body plethysmography depends on Boyle's law
(c) Measurements for the nitrogen washout technique begin at the end of maximal expiration
(d) The helium dilution method only measures communicating gas volume
(e) In a normal adult, body plethysmography overestimates FRC

Answer: a,b,d

Short explanation
Measurements for all techniques begin at the end of normal expiration, as this equals FRC. Both the helium dilution and nitrogen washout techniques only measure ventilating regions of the lung, while body plethysmography measures total volume of gas in the lung. In health, body plethysmography is an accurate measure of FRC.

Long explanation
The functional residual capacity (FRC) is the volume of gas present in the lungs at the end of normal expiration. The FRC cannot be measured using simple spirometry, as it includes the residual volume. It can be measured using helium dilution, multi-breath nitrogen washout or body plethysmography.

The helium dilution technique requires a subject connected to a spirometer containing a known concentration of helium. Starting from the end of normal expiration (i.e. FRC), the subject breathes the gas and the helium distributes between the spirometer, the tubing and the lungs. Once equilibrium is reached, the new concentration of helium is measured. As no helium is lost, due to its low solubility in blood, helium present before equilibrium = helium present after equilibrium:

$$C_1 \times V_{\text{spirometer}} = C_2 \times (V_{\text{spirometer}} + V_{\text{lungs}})$$

where C_1 is the concentration of helium before equilibrium is reached, C_2 is the concentration after equilibrium and V is volume. Rearranging the equation gives

$$V_{\text{lungs}} = V_{\text{spirometer}} \times (C_1 - C_2)/C_2$$

Nitrogen washout measures the elimination of nitrogen from the lungs while the subject breathes 100% oxygen. The test begins from the end of normal expiration and takes place over several minutes. FRC can be calculated, as the concentration originally contained in the FRC was 79%.

Body plethysmography employs an airtight box with the subject sitting inside. At the end of normal expiration, a shutter closes the mouthpiece and the subject makes inspiratory efforts. The volume of the box decreases due to lung expansion and box pressure increases. By applying Boyle's law, the change in lung volume is obtained. Boyle's law is subsequently applied to the gas in the lung, having measured the mouth pressures before and after inspiratory effort, and the FRC is calculated. In a healthy adult, body plethysmography is the most accurate measure of FRC, as it also accounts for gas trapped within the lungs. However, in individuals with severe obstructive lung disease, FRC may be overestimated if the subject experiences acute bronchospasm during testing.

Madama V. *Pulmonary Function Testing and Cardiopulmonary Stress Testing*, 2nd edn. New York, NY: Thomson, 1998; p. 98.

West J. *Respiratory Physiology: the Essentials*, 8th edn. Philadelphia, PA: Lippincott Williams & Wilkins, 2008; pp. 14–16.

Yentis S, Hirsch N, Smith G. *Anaesthesia and Intensive Care A–Z: an Encyclopaedia of Principles and Practice*, 3rd edn. Edinburgh: Butterworth–Heinemann, 2004; pp. 122–3.

MTF Question 57: The Krebs cycle

The citric acid cycle:

(a) Is exclusive to carbohydrate metabolism
(b) Occurs in the cell cytoplasm
(c) Is initiated with citrate as its entry-point substrate
(d) Generates two adenosine triphosphate (ATP) molecules per molecule of glucose
(e) Is an aerobic process

Answer: d,e

Short explanation

The citric acid cycle or Krebs cycle is also known as the tricarboxylic acid (TCA) cycle. The end products of carbohydrate, lipid and protein metabolism enter the citric acid cycle, which is exclusive to the cell mitochondria. Acetyl coenzyme A is the common entry-point substrate initiating the cycle.

Long explanation

The final digestion products of carbohydrate (glucose), lipid (fatty acid) and protein (amino acid) metabolism result in the production of acetyl coenzyme A (acetyl-CoA). This coenzyme is partly derived from one of the B vitamins, panthothenic acid. Acetyl-CoA production yields a small amount of adenosine triphosphate (ATP) energy; however, this coenzyme is the entry-point substrate for the citric acid (Krebs) cycle and subsequent oxidative phosphorylation, which between them generate the majority of the body's energy.

The citric acid cycle is a series of nine biochemical reactions involving several intermediate compounds which undergo decarboxylation and oxidation–reduction reactions in the matrix of the mitochondria. Acetyl-CoA combines with oxaloacetate to form citrate, initiating the cycle's series of reactions. The decarboxylation reactions, resulting from the removal of carbon groups from the intermediate structures, produce the carbon dioxide which is removed via the lungs. The oxidation–reduction reactions produce electron carrier molecules to enter the electron transport chain for the production of further ATP as well as guanosine triphosphate (GTP), which provides the energy for conversion of adenosine diphosphate (ADP) to ATP by substrate-level phosphorylation.

For every glucose molecule (which equates to two acetyl-CoA molecules) entering the cycle six nicotinamide adenine dinucleotide (NADH), two flavin adenine dinucleotide ($FADH_2$), two GTP and six carbon dioxide molecules are produced. This cycle is aerobic and is therefore dependent on the presence of oxygen.

Tortora G J, Grabowski S R. *Principles of Anatomy and Physiology*, 8th edn. New York, NY: HarperCollins, 1996; pp. 818–22.

MTF Question 58: The visual pathway

Regarding the visual pathway:

(a) Axons from the nasal retina decussate in the optic tract
(b) Axons from the temporal retina decussate in the optic chiasm
(c) Axons from the temporal retina synapse in the contralateral lateral geniculate nucleus
(d) The primary visual cortex is located around the calcarine fissure
(e) The optic tracts relay information for eye movement to the superior colliculi

Answer: d,e

Short explanation
Axons derived from the nasal region of the retina decussate in the optic chiasm, while those from the temporal region remain ipsilateral. Hence, the latter synapse in the ipsilateral lateral geniculate nucleus (LGN).

Long explanation
An understanding of the visual pathway is important, as it enables interpretation and management of visual defects. Lesions in the brain can be partially located and identified by mapping these defects. The visual pathway begins as the light hits the photoreceptors on the posterior surface of the retina. The resulting impulses are passed anteriorly to the ganglion cells through a layer of bipolar, horizontal and amacrine cells. From here axons project along the interior surface of the eye, converging to form the optic nerve (CN II) at the 'blind spot'.

The axons arising from the nasal part of the retina cross over (decussate) at the optic chiasm and synapse in the contralateral lateral geniculate nucleus (LGN). The axons arising from the temporal part of the retina remain on the ipsilateral side and synapse into the ipsilateral LGN.

The optic tract consists of optic nerve axons from both the nasal and temporal retina and projects posteriorly on both sides from the optic chiasm to the LGN at the thalamus. From here secondary neurones radiate toward the occipital cortex and the primary visual cortex. This is known as the optic radiation.

The primary visual cortex is located around the calcarine fissure, where the axons from the optic radiation create a topographical projection of the visual field onto the primary visual cortex. As a result, the right primary visual cortex receives visual information from the right temporal retina and the left nasal retina, while the left visual cortex receives information from the left temporal retina and right nasal retina.

The optic tracts also relay impulses to the superior colliculi on the dorsal surface of the brainstem, where it regulates eye movement and posture. It is thought that the visual cortex has three separate regions for interpreting visual information, one for shape, one for colour and one for movement, location and spatial awareness.

Smith T, Pinnock C, Lin T. *Fundamentals of Anaesthesia*, 3rd edn. Cambridge: Cambridge University Press, 2009; p. 405.

MTF Question 59: Resting membrane potential

Regarding the resting membrane potential of cells:

(a) At rest, the cell membrane is more permeable to potassium than sodium
(b) The calculated Nernst potential for chloride is similar to the resting membrane potential

(c) The Nernst equation considers the effect of membrane permeability
(d) The resting membrane potential is less negative in acute potassium deficiency
(e) For nerve cells the resting membrane potential is –90 mV

Answer: a,b

Short explanation

The Nernst equation was modified to account for the importance of selective membrane permeability on determining resting membrane potential, yielding the Goldman–Hodgkin–Katz equation. Hypokalaemia results in a more negative resting membrane potential requiring a greater stimulus to reach the threshold potential and generate an action potential. For nerve cells the resting membrane potential is –70 mV.

Long explanation

The membrane potential occurs because of the differential distribution of charged particles across the cell membrane. This is dependent on the selective membrane permeability to ions and the different ionic concentrations on the inside and outside of cells. Resting cells are relatively permeable to potassium. As the intracellular concentration of potassium is 30 times greater than the extracellular concentration, potassium moves fairly freely down its concentration gradient. However, as potassium moves extracellularly, an electrical gradient is generated opposing the movement of potassium out of the cell. At the resting membrane potential (RMP) the concentration and electrical gradients acting on potassium ions are balanced.

The Nernst equation calculates the potential difference that individual ions would produce if the membrane was freely permeable:

$$E = \frac{RT}{zF} \ln \frac{[\text{ion}]_{\text{out}}}{[\text{ion}]_{\text{in}}} \quad \text{or} \quad E = 58 \, \log_{10} \frac{[\text{ion}]_{\text{out}}}{[\text{ion}]_{\text{in}}} \, \text{mV}$$

where E is the membrane potential in volts, R is the universal gas constant (8.314 J/K per mol), T is the absolute temperature in K, z is the ionic valency of the ion concerned, F is Faraday's constant (96 500 coulombs/mol) and *out* and *in* refer to the extracellular and intracellular concentration of the ion concerned.

For potassium, with an intracellular concentration of 150 mM and an extracellular concentration of 5 mM, the Nernst potential is –90 mV. Since the normal RMP is –70 mV for nerve cells, other ions must contribute to RMP. The cell membrane is moderately permeable to the primary extracellular ion, chloride. The greater extracellular concentration generates a gradient encouraging movement of chloride into the cell. As with potassium, this concentration gradient is balanced by an opposing electrical gradient. The Nernst potential for chloride is –70 mV. Other cations, such as sodium, contribute fairly little to RMP, as cell membrane permeability is low (permeability 100 times less for sodium than for potassium).

The Goldman–Hodgkin–Katz equation accounts for the importance of membrane permeability:

$$E = 58 \, \log_{10} \frac{P_K[K^+]_{\text{out}} + P_{Na}[Na^+]_{\text{out}} + P_{Cl}[Cl^-]_{\text{in}}}{P_K[K^+]_{\text{in}} + P_{Na}[Na^+]_{\text{in}} + P_{Cl}[Cl^-]_{\text{out}}} \, \text{mV}$$

where P is the permeability to each ion.

Given the above equations, it is obvious that a change in extracellular potassium concentration will have an effect on RMP. In potassium deficiency, intra- and extracellular concentrations decrease, although the drop in extracellular potassium is greater. This will result in a more negative resting membrane potential and decreased cell excitability. The opposite is observed with hyperkalaemia. However, both processes lead to muscle weakness.

Power I, Kam P. *Principles of Physiology for the Anaesthetist*. London: Arnold, 2001;
pp. 1–4.
Yentis S, Hirsch N, Smith G. *Anaesthesia and Intensive Care A–Z: an Encyclopaedia of
Principles and Practice*, 3rd edn. Edinburgh: Butterworth–Heinemann, 2004;
pp. 335, 362.

MTF Question 60: Renal blood and plasma flow

Regarding the kidney, which of the following statements are correct?

(a) Renal blood flow can be estimated using para-aminohippuric acid
(b) Approximately 85% of inulin is cleared from the blood during one passage
through the kidney
(c) Renal plasma flow can be estimated using para-aminohippuric acid
(d) The haematocrit must be known to calculate the effective renal plasma flow
(e) Inulin may be used to estimate renal plasma flow

Answer: a,c

Short explanation
Inulin is freely filtered at the glomerulus but is not reabsorbed or secreted. Therefore,
it is a good estimation of the glomerular filtration rate. All of the filtered inulin is
excreted in the urine. However, only 125 mL (25%) of the total renal plasma flow of
600 mL is filtered by the kidney each minute. The haematocrit is required to calculate
the renal blood flow.

Long explanation
Clearance is defined as the volume of plasma (in mL) completely cleared of a substance
per minute by an organ. For the kidney, the clearance of a substance is:

$$\text{Clearance}_x \ (\text{mL/min}) = \frac{U_x V}{P_x}$$

where U_x is the urine concentration of x (mmol/L), P_x is the plasma concentration of x
(mmol/L) and V is the urine flow (mL/min). Para-aminohippuric acid (PAH) is an
organic acid that is used as an estimation of renal plasma flow (RPF). It is incompletely
filtered at the glomerulus but also secreted from the peritubular capillaries into the
proximal tubules. When the PAH blood concentration is less than the tubular maximum (10 mg/100 mL plasma), all of the plasma perfusing the filtering and secreting
parts of the kidney is completely cleared of PAH. A normal value for renal plasma flow
is 600 mL/min

$$\text{RPF} \ (\text{mL/min}) = \frac{U_{\text{PAH}} V}{P_{\text{PAH}}}$$

If the haematocrit is known, renal blood flow (RBF) may be estimated using the
following equation:

$$\text{RBF} \ (\text{mL/min}) = \frac{\text{RPF}}{(1 - \text{haematocrit})}$$

At rest, the total renal blood flow is approximately 1100 mL/min. PAH extraction from
renal blood is only about 90% following one passage through the kidney, as not all
blood passes through the glomerulus or peritubular capillaries (some perfuses the
perirenal fat and medulla).

Smith T, Pinnock C, Lin T. *Fundamentals of Anaesthesia*, 3rd edn. Cambridge: Cambridge University Press, 2009; pp. 331–2.

Yentis S, Hirsch N, Smith G. *Anaesthesia and Intensive Care A–Z: an Encyclopaedia of Principles and Practice*, 3rd edn. Edinburgh: Butterworth-Heinemann, 2004; p. 450.

SBA Question 61: Cellular respiration

A healthy 30-year-old runs the London Marathon. Immediately after completing the race serum lactate levels are measured and found to be 8.8 mmol/L. During exercise cellular respiration is both aerobic and anaerobic, leading to a build-up of lactate. Which ONE of the following processes in cellular respiration consumes oxygen?

(a) Metabolism of glucose to glucose-6-phosphate
(b) Metabolism of phosphoenol pyruvate to pyruvate
(c) Formation of acetyl-CoA from pyruvate and coenzyme A
(d) Formation of lactate from pyruvate
(e) Formation of water at the end of the electron transport chain

Answer: e

Short explanation

For efficient production of energy, oxygen is required. In the three processes glycolysis, the citric acid cycle and oxidative phosphorylation, oxygen is not consumed until the last stage of oxidative phosphorylation. Glycolysis will continue in the absence of oxygen, but the citric acid cycle and oxidative phosphorylation do require the presence of oxygen.

Long explanation

Production of energy in the form of adenosine triphosphate (ATP) from carbohydrates is most efficient in the presence of oxygen. There are three basic pathways occurring in cells. Glycolysis occurs in the cellular cytoplasm and is independent of oxygen, while the citric acid cycle (Krebs cycle) and oxidative phosphorylation take place in mitochondria and only proceed in the presence of oxygen. Aerobic respiration is the most efficient way to produce ATP, forming 38 molecules for each mole of glucose. Anaerobic respiration yields only two molecules of ATP.

Glycolysis breaks down glucose to pyruvate in a series of 10 reactions of which glucose to glucose-6-phosphate is the first and phosphoenol pyruvate to pyruvate is the last. This process requires two molecules of ATP but also produces four molecules (net gain of two). No oxygen is utilised and no carbon dioxide is produced, but one molecule of NAD^+ (an electron carrier) is utilised. In the absence of oxygen, pyruvate is metabolised into lactate; this process regenerates the electron carrier (NADH + H to NAD^+) allowing glycolysis to continue, which means that two molecules of ATP per mole of glucose continue to be produced, but lactate will build up in the cell.

One of the steps in the citric acid cycle is the formation of acetyl coenzyme A (acetyl-CoA). The citric acid cycle does not use oxygen, but can only take place in aerobic conditions as the process utilises NAD^+ and these molecules must be regenerated in oxidative phosphorylation for the cycle to continue. The cycle consists of multiple steps producing electrons that are transferred to high energy carriers (NADH + H and $FADH_2$) to transport them to the electron transfer chains for oxidative phosphorylation.

The electrons from the citric acid cycle enter the electron transport chain (a series of cytochromes) and are transported along it, releasing energy. The energy is used to pump hydrogen ions against their concentration gradient. At three points along the chain are pores allowing hydrogen ions to flow along the concentration gradient, and energy released from this flow forms ATP from ADP + Pi. At the end of the chain oxygen reacts with the remaining hydrogen ions (from NADH + H and FADH$_2$) and electrons to form water:

$$2e^- + 1/2\ O_2 + 2H = 2H_2O$$

Power I, Kam P. *Principles of Physiology for the Anaesthetist*. London: Arnold, 2001; pp. 65–7.

SBA Question 62: Gas flow measurement

Which one of the following is NOT used to measure gas flow?

(a) Rotameter
(b) Pitot tube pneumotachograph
(c) Wright respirometer
(d) Wright peak flowmeter
(e) Fleisch pneumotachograph

Answer: c

Short explanation

The Wright respirometer is an expiratory volume recorder that uses gas flow to spin a vane to measure volume. All the rest measure gas flow.

Long explanation

There are many different ways of measuring gas flow and volume. Volume and flow are related: if the volume of fluid passing a point can be measured over a given time then the flow can be calculated. As gases are compressible, there are specific problems associated with the measurement of gas flows and volumes that are not present when measuring liquids. The following are used for gas flow measurement:

- A rotameter – variable-orifice, constant-pressure flowmeter. It consists of a tapered glass tube containing a bobbin. The bobbin is supported in the tapered tube by gas flow and, as the flow increases, the bobbin rises in the tube. There is a variable orifice around the bobbin that depends on the gas flow. The pressure across the bobbin remains constant. There is a mixture of laminar and turbulent flow, so calibration depends on both the density and the viscosity of the gas.
- A Wright peak flowmeter – variable-orifice flowmeter. This uses rotation of a vane to open a circular slot, allowing gas to escape, opposed by a force from a coiled spring. A pointer mounted on the vane registers the movement on a calibrated dial.
- A mass flowmeter – electric current passes through a thermistor, the resistance of which varies with temperature. It aims to keep the temperature of the thermistor constant as gas flows over it and extracts heat energy. The current required to keep the temperature constant is a measure of gas flow.
- A pneumotachograph – constant-orifice, variable-pressure flowmeter. It is used in anaesthetic circuits and causes little resistance to gas flow. There are several types including the screen, Fleisch, hot-wire and modified Pitot tube pneumotachograph.

The Wright respirometer is an expiratory volume recorder that uses gas flow to spin a vane to measure volume. It can be used to measure tidal volume in anaesthesia. Volume measurement is achieved by monitoring the continuous rotation of a vane as it is moved by the flow of gas. The vane does not rotate when the gas flow is reversed.

It is calibrated for use for tidal volume measurement and is inaccurate if it is used to measure a continuous flow.

Davis PD, Kenny GNC. *Basic Physics and Measurement in Anaesthesia*, 5th edn. Oxford: Butterworth–Heinemann, 2003; pp. 25–31.

SBA Question 63: Bupivacaine pKa

During an in-theatre discussion with a consultant about the relevance of pKa, you are asked the following question. The pKa of lidocaine is 7.9, and at a pH of 7.4, 75% of the drug is ionised. The pKa of bupivacaine is 8.1. What percentage of bupivacaine is un-ionised at a pH of 7.4?

(a) 42%
(b) 37%
(c) 33%
(d) 26%
(e) 17%

Answer: e

Short explanation
As bupivicaine has a higher pKa than lidocaine, at physiological pH bupivicaine will be relatively less un-ionised than lidocaine

Long explanation
This question can be worked out with basic knowledge without even having to complete the formula and calculate the inverse log. We know that local anaesthetics work less well in infected acid tissue because they are more ionised at the lower pH and therefore less able to enter the neurones and have an action. All local anaesthetics are weak bases.

We know that lidocaine is heavily ionised at low pH, 75% ionised at pH 7.4 and 50% ionised at pH 7.9, because the pKa is the pH at which 50% of a drug is ionised and 50% is un-ionised.

Bupivacaine has a pKa of 8.1 and so will have to get to a relatively higher pH before becoming as un-ionised as lidocaine. Their pKa values are not wildly apart so you would therefore expect bupivacaine to be marginally less un-ionised than lidocaine at pH 7.4. However, if you want to do the calculations, at a pH of 7.4:

$$pH = pK_a + log\left(\frac{[B]}{[BH^+]}\right)$$

$$7.4 = 8.1 + log\left(\frac{[B]}{[BH^+]}\right)$$

$$-0.7 = log\left(\frac{[B]}{[BH^+]}\right)$$

$$0.1995 = \left(\frac{[B]}{[BH^+]}\right)$$

Peck T, Hill S, Williams M. *Pharmacology for Anaesthesia and Intensive Care*, 3rd edn. Cambridge: Cambridge University Press, 2008; p. 166.

SBA Question 64: Anaesthetic equipment checklist

The Association of Anaesthetists of Great Britain and Ireland (AAGBI) produced a checklist for anaesthetic equipment in 2004. As recommended by AAGBI, which of the following checks comes first?

(a) Check with a 'tug test' that each pipeline is correctly inserted into the appropriate gas supply terminal
(b) Check the breathing system to be employed
(c) Check all monitoring devices, particularly the oxygen analyser
(d) Check that alternative means to ventilate the patient is immediately available
(e) Check the operation of the flowmeters

Answer: c

Short explanation

The AAGBI checklist is an 11-point checklist that should be used to check the anaesthetic machine prior to anaesthetising any case. The full checklist should be available on all anaesthetic machines.

Long explanation

It is a mandatory procedure to check anaesthetic equipment prior to its use. A major contributory cause of anaesthetic misadventures, resulting at worst in hypoxic brain damage or death, has been the use of anaesthetic machines and/or breathing systems which had not been adequately checked beforehand by an anaesthetist. It is the responsibility of all NHS trusts to ensure that all personnel are trained in the use and checking of relevant equipment.

The checking procedure is applicable to all anaesthetic machines, should take only a few minutes to perform, and represents an important aspect of patient safety. There should be a record kept with the anaesthetic machine documenting each check done.

The checking procedure covers all aspects of the anaesthetic delivery system from the gas supply pipelines to the machine and breathing systems, including filters, connectors and airway devices. It includes an outline check for ventilators, suction, monitoring and ancillary equipment. Of note, the oxygen failure alarm must be checked on a weekly basis by disconnecting the oxygen hose while the oxygen flowmeter is turned on. In addition to sounding an alarm, which must sound for at least 7 seconds, oxygen failure warning devices are also linked to a gas shut-off device. Anaesthetists must be aware both of the tone of the alarm and also what gases will continue to flow with the make of anaesthetic machine in use.

When checking the breathing system, the anaesthetist must ensure the correct configuration and firm attachment of all connections. For the coaxial breathing system, the inner tube must be checked. This can be done with Pethick's test, which involves closing the expiratory valve and filling the reservoir bag by occluding the distal end of the tubing. The oxygen flush should now be used with the tube unobstructed, and the bag should empty due to gas entrainment, providing the inner tube is not detached.

All anaesthetists should be familiar with the checklist guidelines, and the use of checklists and associated procedures is an integral part of training in anaesthesia. As such, it forms part of the Royal College of Anaesthetists' Competency Based Training.

Recommendations from AAGBI are available online at www.aagbi.org/publications/publications-guidelines (accessed 15 March 2012).
Yentis S, Hirsch N, Smith G. *Anaesthesia and Intensive Care A–Z: an Encyclopaedia of Principles and Practice*, 4th edn. Edinburgh: Butterworth–Heinemann, 2009; p. 111.

SBA Question 65: Renal excretion of drugs

In a patient on haemodialysis secondary to end-stage renal failure, which of the following drugs requires the least significant dose adjustment?

(a) Rifampicin
(b) Flucloxacillin
(c) Lithium
(d) Ranitidine
(e) Pancuronium

Answer: a

Short explanation

All the drugs are excreted largely unchanged, but rifampicin is highly lipid-soluble and is excreted in the bile. Flucloxacillin and ranitidine are actively secreted in the proximal tubule, while lithium and pancuronium are passively filtered because of their permanent charge.

Long explanation

The kidney is the major site of drug excretion for the body. The majority of drugs which are < 30 000 kDa in size are excreted in the urine, with the bile being the second most common site. Drugs are more likely to be excreted unchanged in the urine if they are small, ionised or otherwise water-soluble and not extensively protein-bound.

The majority of drugs are metabolised prior to excretion, but all the listed drugs undergo metabolism only to a minor degree. Flucloxacillin and ranitidine are secreted in the proximal tubule, but pancuronium and lithium (which both have a permanent charge) are freely filtered into the glomerular ultrafiltrate and thence excreted. Rifampicin is highly lipid-soluble and primarily excreted unchanged into the bile. The active transport mechanisms that facilitate this excretion can be saturated in high dose, in which case some drug is excreted unchanged in the urine, but this will not exceed 80% of the dose.

Peck T, Hill S, Williams M. *Pharmacology for Anaesthesia and Intensive Care*, 3rd edn. Cambridge: Cambridge University Press, 2008.

SBA Question 66: Bohr equation

A significant reduction in physiological dead space occurs in a number of disease states. Which of the following equations best describes measurement of physiological dead space? (V_D = volume of dead space, V_T = tidal volume, P_ACO_2 = alveolar partial pressure of CO_2, $PaCO_2$ = arterial partial pressure of CO_2, P_ECO_2 = mixed expired partial pressure of CO_2)

(a) $\dfrac{V_T}{V_D} = \dfrac{P_ACO_2 - P_ECO_2}{PaCO_2}$

(b) $\dfrac{V_D}{V_T} = \dfrac{P_ECO_2 - P_ACO_2}{P_ECO_2}$

(c) $\dfrac{V_D}{V_T} = \dfrac{P_ACO_2 - P_ECO_2}{P_ACO_2}$

(d) $\dfrac{V_T}{V_D} = \dfrac{P_aCO_2 - P_ECO_2}{P_aCO_2}$

(e) $\dfrac{V_D}{V_T} = \dfrac{P_aCO_2 - P_ECO_2}{P_aCO_2}$

Answer: c

Short explanation
Physiological dead space is commonly measured using the Bohr equation. The ratio of dead space to tidal volume is quoted as a ratio and is derived from the fractional difference between P_ACO_2 and P_ECO_2.

Long explanation
The Bohr equation is used to derive physiological dead space. The final equation quoted in the third option is derived from a long sequence of shuffling parameters. An important statement to make when explaining the Bohr equation is that all expired CO_2 is equal to the inspired CO_2 plus the CO_2 excreted from the lungs. Dead space is the volume of gas that does eliminate CO_2. The concentration of CO_2 in inspired gas is minimal, so it can be ignored. The following sequence explains how the Bohr equation is derived.

V_T = tidal volume, V_D = volume of dead space, V_A = volume of alveolar component
F_E = fractional concentration of CO_2 in expired gas
F_A = fractional concentration of CO_2 in alveolar gas
$V_T \times F_E = V_A \times F_A$
If $V_T = V_A + V_D$, then $V_A = V_T - V_D$
By substituting V_A into the first equation, then $V_T \times F_E = (V_T - V_D) \times F_A$
Which is therefore equal to $V_T \times F_E = (V_T \times F_A) - (V_D \times F_A)$

By further rearrangement:

$$\frac{V_D}{V_T} = \frac{F_A - F_E}{F_A}$$

By using Dalton's law of partial pressure, the partial pressure of CO_2 is proportional to its concentration, therefore:

$$\frac{V_D}{V_T} = \frac{P_ACO_2 - P_ECO_2}{P_ACO_2}$$

Arterial CO_2 tension is easier to measure that alveolar tension, and arterial CO_2 is virtually the same as the arterial tension, therefore:

$$\frac{V_D}{V_T} = \frac{PaCO_2 - P_ECO_2}{PaCO_2}$$

The normal value for dead space to tidal volume ratio during resting breathing is between 0.2 and 0.35. Alternative methods of measuring dead space include the 'Koulouris' technique. This method is non-invasive and analysis is based on expired carbon dioxide volume versus expired tidal volume from a single expiration. It remains to be fully validated.

Erdemli G. Lecture notes on human respiratory system physiology; pp. 11–13. Available online at www.liv.ac.uk/~gdwill/hons/gul_lect.pdf (accessed 15 March 2012).

Tang Y, Turner MJ, Baker AB. Effects of alveolar dead-space, shunt and distribution on respiratory dead-space measurements. *Br J Anaesth* 2005; **95**: 538–48. Available online at bja.oxfordjournals.org/content/95/4/538 (accessed 15 March 2012).

West JB. *Respiratory Physiology*, 7th edn. Philadelphia, PA: Lippincott Williams & Wilkins. 2005; pp. 19–21.

SBA Question 67: Temperature measurement

An 80-year-old gentleman is booked for an elective laparotomy. During your preoperative assessment you identify the need for careful temperature regulation during the procedure. Which of the following sites for temperature measurement would be the most accurate indirect measure of cerebral temperature for this patient?

(a) The rectum
(b) The nasal passage
(c) Peripheral skin
(d) The lower oesophagus
(e) The nasopharynx

Answer: d

Short explanation

Rectal temperature varies because of the presence of gut flora, faeces and blood flow from the lower limbs. Peripheral skin temperature may vary considerably from core temperature. Ambient temperature affects both nasal passage and nasopharyngeal temperature measurement to a greater degree than lower oesophageal temperature measurement.

Long explanation

Sites commonly used for temperature measurement to represent core temperature include oesophageal, nasopharynx, tympanic membrane, blood, bladder and rectal.

- Oesophageal temperature should be taken from the lower third of the oesophagus, and it provides a good estimate of cerebral blood temperature. Placed above this level, the probe may under-read due to cooling from inspired gases.
- The nasopharyngeal temperature probe is placed just behind the soft palate and is less accurate then the oesophageal temperature as a representation of core temperature but is more accessible.
- The tympanic membrane provides an accurate representation of hypothalamic temperature. It is less invasive, has a short response time and correlates well with oesophageal temperature, but it does not allow continuous measurements.
- Blood temperature can be measured using a pulmonary artery flotation catheter and is the best continuous measurement of core temperature.
- Rectal temperature is influenced by heat generated from gut flora, the cooling effect of blood returning from the lower limbs and the insulation of the probe by faeces. It is normally about 0.5–1.0 °C higher than core temperature and has a slow response time.

Temperature gradients exist between different sites of the body, and this can be useful in clinical practice. The gradient between a skin temperature and a core temperature can be used as a marker of peripheral perfusion.

Smith T, Pinnock C, Lin T. *Fundamentals of Anaesthesia*, 3rd edn. Cambridge: Cambridge University Press, 2009; pp. 822–3.
Yentis S, Hirsch N, Smith G. *Anaesthesia and Intensive Care A–Z: an Encyclopaedia of Principles and Practice*, 4th edn. Edinburgh: Butterworth–Heinemann, 2009; p. 504.

SBA Question 68: Breathing system filters

Breathing system filters (BSFs) act as a barrier, protecting patients from particles and pathogens entering the respiratory system. Which one of the following is NOT a recognised mechanism used in BSFs?

(a) Interception
(b) Inertial impaction
(c) Electrostatic repulsion
(d) Diffusion
(e) Gravitational settling

Answer: c

Short explanation

There are five major filtration mechanisms that explain how BSFs work. These are interception, inertial impaction, diffusion, gravitational settling and electrostatic attraction (not electrostatic repulsion). Which is the most effective depends to a large extent on the size of the particles to be filtered.

Long explanation

BSFs are designed to replace the filtering function of the nasopharynx, reducing contamination of anaesthetic breathing equipment (so allowing its use between patients), and they also have a role in warming and humidification. BSFs reduce the passage of gas-borne particles by five mechanisms: interception, inertial impaction, diffusion, gravitational settling and electrostatic attraction. How effective these mechanisms are depends on the size of the particle passing through the BSF.

Depending on the type of filter there is a particular size of particle, known as the 'most penetrating particle size' (PPS), which will pass through it most easily. The PPS usually measures in the range of 0.05–0.5 µm in diameter. For particles around this size the two most important filtration mechanisms are diffusion and interception. With interception, any particles in the gas stream coming within a one-particle radius of the surface of the BSF fibres will be trapped. With diffusion, particles undergoing Brownian motion cross gas streams, so increasing the probability of them striking a BSF fibre. For large particles in slow-moving air, gravitational settling allows the BSF fibres to trap them.

Inertial impaction occurs when a particle is so large that it is unable to adjust quickly to the abrupt changes in gas-stream direction near a filter. The particle, because of its inertia, will continue along its original path and hit the filter. This type of filtration mechanism is predominant when high gas velocity and/or dense packing of the filter media is present.

Electrostatic attraction works for both charged particles (most gas-borne particulate material carries some electrostatic charge) and neutral particles. The former are attracted to oppositely charged fibres within the BSF by coulombic attraction (the force of attraction between positive and negative particles) and the latter are attracted to charged fibres within a BSF.

Wilkes AR. Breathing system filters. *Br J Anaesth CEPD Rev* 2002; **2**: 151–4. Available online at ceaccp.oxfordjournals.org/content/2/5/151 (accessed 15 March 2012).

SBA Question 69: Defibrillation

Regarding the defibrillator, which ONE of the following statements is most correct?

(a) Stored energy can be calculated by ½ charge (millicoulombs) multiplied by the potential (volts)

(b) The coulomb is the capacitance of an object for which the electrical potential increases by one volt when one coulomb of charge is added to it

(c) Stored energy can be calculated by ½ charge (millicoulombs) divided by the potential (volts)

(d) The farad is the quantity of electric charge that passes some point when a current of one ampere flows for a period of one second

(e) The capacitor functions to smooth out the energy delivered to the patient

Answer: a

Short explanation

The farad is the capacitance of an object for which the electrical potential increases by one volt when one coulomb of charge is added to it. The coulomb is the quantity of electric charge that passes some point when a current of one ampere flows for a period of one second. The inductor functions to smooth out the energy delivered to the patient.

Long explanation

The defibrillator is used in the treatment of ventricular fibrillation and is an example of an instrument that stores electric charge and then releases it in a controlled fashion. The key component is the capacitor, which consists of two plates separated by an insulator, with a potential difference of up to 8000 V between its plates. The stored charge is then released during discharge; this is proportional to the potential difference.

Up to 400 J is used for external defibrillation, although only about 360 J is actually delivered to the patient because of internal energy loss. Thoracic impedance is reduced by the first shock, so a second discharge at the same level will deliver greater energy to the heart.

An inductor, included in the output circuit, lengthens the duration of the current pulse. When charging, a switch is activated so that the current from the mains flows to the capacitor. This then charges in an exponential manner. When the discharge switch is activated, current from the capacitor flows via the inductor to the pads.

Stored energy can be calculated by ½ charge (millicoulombs) multiplied by the potential (volts). For example, if the defibrillator is on its maximum setting and a potential of 5000 V is applied across the two plates of the capacitor, an equivalent of 160 millicoulombs of charge is produced. Therefore the stored charge will equal ½ × 160 × 5000, which will give 400 J.

A monophasic defibrillator produces a single pulse of current in one direction across the chest, whereas a biphasic defibrillator produces two consecutive pulses. The latter produces a lower defibrillation threshold and therefore is more efficient.

Davis PD, Kenny GNC. *Basic Physics and Measurement in Anaesthesia*, 5th edn. Oxford: Butterworth–Heinemann, 2003; pp. 157–9.

Yentis S, Hirsch N, Smith G. *Anaesthesia and Intensive Care A–Z: an Encyclopaedia of Principles and Practice*, 4th edn. Edinburgh: Butterworth – Heinemann, 2009; p. 155.

SBA Question 70: Hypotension on ICU

A 73-year-old, 61 kg female patient is admitted, intubated, to ICU following an aspiration of gastric contents post induction of anaesthesia. She is hypoxic with a PaO_2 of 6.1 kPa on FiO_2 of 1.0. She has had fluid boluses, metaraminol boluses, and now a noradrenaline infusion to manage worsening hypotension. You insert your cardiac output monitoring device and note the following data: heart rate 96 beats/min, blood pressure 68/46 mmHg, cardiac output 2.5 L/min, pulmonary capillary wedge pressure 20 mmHg, systemic vascular resistance 1400 dyn·s/cm^5. The ONE agent to best normalise this patient's haemodynamic variables would be:

(a) Noradrenaline
(b) Adrenaline
(c) Dobutamine
(d) Vasopressin
(e) Levosimendan

Answer: c

Short explanation
This patient is well filled, vasoconstricted and has a poor cardiac output. She would be normalised by an inotrope and a dilator, which fits the profile for dobutamine.

Long explanation
This patient has tachycardia with severe hypotension but appears to be adequately filled with intravenous fluid. Her haemodynamics indicate low cardiac output with high systemic vascular resistance. She is vasoconstricted, with inadequate left ventricular function. She would benefit from an inotrope and a vasodilator.

Dobutamine is an inodilator and would probably be the agent of choice here. Both adrenaline and noradrenaline are likely to worsen the vasoconstriction. Vasopressin (antidiuretic hormone, ADH) is principally of use when vasoconstriction is required. Relative vasopressin deficiency occurs during advanced shock, and vascular beds may not be able to vasodilate or vasoconstrict in their normal physiological way any more. Vasopressin seems to restore this capacity and has been principally used in advanced septic or hypovolaemic shock. Levosimendan is an inodilator but is not recommended in severe hypotension.

SBA Question 71: Cardiac axis

A 25-year-old woman who is 16 weeks pregnant is admitted to hospital with sudden onset of breathlessness and collapse. A transthoracic echocardiogram suggests a massive pulmonary embolus. An ECG is studied and shows sinus tachycardia with right axis deviation. The cardiac axis is likely to lie at which of these angles?

(a) −60 degrees
(b) +60 degrees
(c) +90 degrees
(d) +120 degrees
(e) −90 degrees

Answer: d

Short explanation
The cardiac axis points to the average spread of ventricular depolarisation. Displacement of the axis from a normal range of −30° to +90° can be a useful indication of pathology. Right axis deviation lies beyond +90°.

Long explanation
The cardiac axis points to the average spread of ventricular depolarisation. Displacement of the axis from a normal range of −30° to +90° can be a useful indication of pathology.

There are a number of methods to calculate the cardiac axis. The axis points in the direction where the upward deflection (R wave) is larger than the downward deflection (S wave). The limb leads look at the heart from different directions and can be used to determine the angle of the cardiac axis. The point at which the R wave equals the S wave in a particular lead indicates that the axis points 90° angle away from it.

Lead I lies at 0°, lead II at +60°, lead aVF at +90°, lead III at +120°, aVR at −150° and aVL at −30° (see diagram).

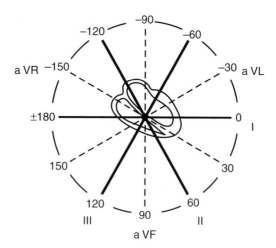

Hampton J R. *The ECG Made Easy*, 7th edn. Edinburgh: Churchill Livingstone, 2008.

SBA Question 72: Treating dehydration

You are working as a ship's doctor in the tropics. The ship rescues a 40-year-old, 72 kg man from an island who was shipwrecked 2 days previously. He has had nothing to eat or drink for 2 days and the average daytime temperature has been 34 °C. He looks severely dehydrated but is conscious and cooperative. Which ONE of the following would be your fluid resuscitation of choice over the next 24 hours?

(a) Let him drink water freely
(b) Cautiously allow to drink water and administer 2000 mL of 5% dextrose solution intravenously over the next 24 hours
(c) Cautiously allow to drink water and administer 3000 mL of Hartmann's solution intravenously over the next 24 hours
(d) Prohibit oral fluids and administer 4000 mL of 0.9% saline solution intravenously over the next 24 hours
(e) Prohibit oral fluids and administer 5000 mL of dextrose saline solution intravenously over the next 24 hours

Answer: c

Short explanation
This man is conscious and cooperative, and so is best managed with oral fluid and electrolytes. The only option providing this is the Hartmann's solution.

Long explanation
After 2 days at 34 °C without food or drink, this man will be severely dehydrated and probably also suffering heatstroke. He will be in a substantial net deficit of both water and electrolytes and will need replacement of both.

Mild dehydration presents with thirst, orthostatic hypotension, lethargy and fatigueability. Mild dehydration symptoms are seen with the dehydration people experience in their everyday lives, equating to a 1–2% water deficit. As dehydration worsens, oliguria may develop along with tachycardia, tachypnoea, rising body temperature due to absence of sweating, headaches, nausea and confusion. This typically is seen as 5% water deficit approaches. At 10% deficit, spasticity of muscles and loss of vision is reported, with unconsciousness also likely. Dehydration at 15% is often fatal.

This man is described as severely dehydrated but is still conscious and cooperative. Oral fluid resuscitation is appropriate and recommended, although it may not be adequate alone. An oral balanced salt and sugar rehydration fluid would be ideal. However, oral water would be inadvisable as it will not provide the required electrolytes. The same would also be true of the intravenous 5% dextrose solution. The option of oral intake and Hartmann's solution would be an acceptable starting plan, although this would ideally require regular monitoring of clinical condition and investigative monitoring of plasma electrolytes and glucose.

A widely used plan for dehydrated patients is to administer half their deficit in the first 24 hours. Considering additional losses such as from sweating in this scenario, the volume of fluid in the Hartmann's option may therefore be inadequate, depending on the volume taken orally, and would require regular monitoring.

SBA Question 73: Hypotension during laparotomy

You are required to take over an emergency laparotomy in a 54-year-old, 80 kg male patient with a history of well-controlled hypertension who is otherwise previously fit and well. You insert an oesophageal Doppler probe and note the following haemodynamic observations: heart rate 103 beats/min, blood pressure 74/49 mmHg, cardiac output 4.1 L/min, flow time corrected (FTc) 290 milliseconds. Your initial management should be ONE of the following:

(a) Give a 200 mL intravenous colloid bolus over 5 minutes
(b) Give a 200 mL intravenous colloid bolus over 5 minutes and start an intravenous infusion of dobutamine
(c) Give a 200 mL intravenous colloid bolus over 5 minutes and start an intravenous infusion of metaraminol
(d) Give a 200 mL intravenous colloid bolus over 5 minutes and start an intravenous infusion of noradrenaline
(e) Start an intravenous infusion of glyceryl trinitrate

Answer: a

Short explanation
The haemodynamic measurements would indicate hypovolaemia. Rule out pure hypovolaemia as a cause of low pressure to avoid administering inotropes and vasoconstrictors to an empty circulation.

Long explanation
The haemodynamic measurements of a tachycardia and hypotension with a low(ish) cardiac output would indicate hypovolaemia. This should be ruled out before giving vasoactive drugs, as one of the reasons for side effects such as peripheral circulatory shutdown from such drugs follows administration to an underfilled circulation. Hypovolaemia needs to be ruled out first, and there is nothing to indicate that this is anything other than hypovolaemia.

The FTc would also indicate this is the case. The FTc is the duration of the peak on the Doppler trace corrected to a heart rate of 60 beats per minute and is an indication of left ventricular filling and afterload. The normal range is 330–360 milliseconds, and it correlates inversely with systemic vascular resistance.

The best plan would be to give a rapid colloid fluid bolus and reassess the haemodynamic state. Adding a vasoactive agent can wait until the response to an intravenous bolus is assessed. Coincident administration would make the subsequent diagnostic process, particularly interpretation of the Doppler data, difficult.

SBA Question: 74: Cardiovascular effects of IPPV

During transfer of a ventilated patient to a regional neurosurgical unit there are several periods of cardiovascular instability requiring titration of the infusion of vasoactive medication. Which of the following statements is NOT a plausible explanation for the cardiovascular instability encountered during intermittent positive-pressure ventilation (IPPV)?

(a) Inspiration produces a decrease in venous return
(b) Inspiration produces an increase in left ventricular filling
(c) Right atrial compression produces a decrease in venous return
(d) Expiration produces an increase in right ventricular filling
(e) The secretion of atrial natriuretic peptide is reduced

Answer: e

Short explanation
There is an increase in the production of atrial natriuretic peptide (ANP) during mechanical ventilation. The decrease in venous return means that the atria do not distend as much, so the volume receptors are not activated and production of ANP therefore decreases.

Long explanation
There are a number of multisystem physiological effects of intermittent positive-pressure ventilation (IPPV). The cardiovascular effects are mainly caused by the increase in intrathoracic pressure causing pressure changes on the heart, great vessels and vascular bed within the thorax. The most significant change is the reduction in venous return, which is mainly caused by right atrial compression, and this is dependent on the increase in pleural pressure.

The pleural and airway pressures both increase with IPPV, and the difference between the two pressures is termed 'transmural pressure'. Lung and chest wall compliance values are important in determining how much of the airway pressure is transmitted to the pleural space. The lung and chest wall compliances are almost equal, so the transmural pressure is equal to the change in pleural pressure in normal lungs. If a high tidal volume is set, the lung compliance will be high and chest wall compliance will be low, which will cause the pressure increase to be exaggerated.

During inspiration the intrathoracic pressure increases, causing a reduction in right ventricular preload because right atrial compression impedes venous return. Conversely, left ventricular preload increases during the inspiratory phase because blood is squeezed out of the pulmonary capillary bed. The intrathoracic pressure decreases on expiration, allowing an increase in right ventricular filling. At functional residual capacity (FRC), the right ventricular afterload is usually minimal (equal to the pulmonary vascular resistance).

In normal lungs, mechanical inspiration causes dilation of the large blood vessels, but the small alveolar blood vessels become compressed so there is minimal overall change in pulmonary vascular resistance. In patients with hyperinflated lungs or with large amounts of applied positive end-expiratory pressure (PEEP), the increase in lung volume may substantially increase the right ventricular afterload.

A tutorial on setting up IPPV is available online at www.ccmtutorials.com/rs/mv/ strategy (accessed 15 March 2012).

SBA Question 75: Pulse oximetry

You devise a new cardiovascular monitor that requires light to be shone through blood at two different wavelengths at which absorption of light is unaffected by the relative proportions of oxyhaemoglobin and deoxyhaemoglobin. Which ONE of the following combinations of light wavelengths would be best?

(a) 545 nm and 850 nm
(b) 530 nm and 815 nm
(c) 585 nm and 855 nm
(d) 570 nm and 905 nm
(e) 590 nm and 805 nm

Answer: e

Short explanation
An isobestic point is the specific wavelength at which two chemical species have the same molar absorptivity. For oxyhaemoglobin and deoxyhaemoglobin the two points are at 590 nm and 805 nm

Long explanation
An isobestic point is defined as the wavelength at which substances absorb the same amount of light (i.e. they have the same molar absorptivity, ε). Oxyhaemoglobin and deoxyhaemoglobin share two isobestic points, one at 590 nm and one at 805 nm. These points may be used as reference points in pulse oximeters, as it is only at these points that light absorption is independent of saturation. Some early oximeters corrected for haemoglobin concentration by using these isobestic points.

For substances to share an isobestic point the relationship between their extinction coefficients (how strongly a substance absorbs light at a given wavelength) must be a linear one. This makes the possibility of more than two substances sharing an isobestic point extremely unlikely, as they would all need to have the same extinction coefficients; otherwise, as concentration varied the relationship would be lost and the isobestic point would be lost.

SBA Question 76: Causes of ventilatory failure

Which of the following conditions is most likely to cause respiratory failure secondary to hypoventilation?

(a) Acute respiratory distress syndrome
(b) Acute exacerbation of asthma with peak expiratory flow rate 60% of that predicted
(c) Aspiration pneumonitis
(d) Acute inflammatory demyelinating polyneuropathy
(e) Acute pulmonary embolus

Answer: d

Short explanation

Acute respiratory distress syndrome (ARDS), aspiration pneumonitis and acute pulmonary embolus more typically cause respiratory failure secondary to either ventilation/perfusion mismatch or shunt if severe. Patients usually hyperventilate with acute exacerbation of asthma where peak expiratory flow rate is 60% of that predicted.

Long explanation

Hypoventilation is effectively reduced alveolar ventilation due to either a reduction in respiratory rate or a reduction in tidal volume or both. Hypoventilation is caused either by a reduction in central respiratory drive or by a physical impairment to breathing.

Opioids are a common cause of decreased respiratory drive. An example of a physical impairment to breathing is acute inflammatory demyelinating polyneuropathy (otherwise known as Guillain–Barré syndrome). This is a bilaterally symmetrical ascending peripheral demyelinating neuropathy and easily impairs transmission of the nerves supplying the muscles that are involved in coordinating breathing.

Inadequate ventilatory effort leads to inadequate gas exchange, so there is a build-up in alveolar CO_2, which causes an increase in the arterial CO_2 tension ($PaCO_2$).

The resulting hypercapnia is usually accompanied by hypoxia because of a shift in the balance of the alveolar gas equation if supplementary oxygen is not provided. If alveolar ventilation is halved, then $PaCO_2$ doubles once steady state has been reached. If there is a sudden increase in alveolar ventilation after a steady period (at least several hours) of hypoventilation, then the alveolar O_2 and CO_2 tensions take time to re-set. The alveolar, and hence arterial, CO_2 tension takes longer because of the large CO_2 stores within the body (bicarbonate and carbamino compounds).

Kaynar AM, Sharma S. Respiratory failure. *Medscape Reference* 2012. Available online at emedicine.medscape.com/article/167981 (accessed 15 March 2012).
Ventilatery failure. *Merck Manual*. Available online at www.merck.com/mmpe/sec06/ch065/ch065d.html (accessed 15 March 2010).

SBA Question 77: Fentanyl patch dose equivalent

A patient arrives at preoperative assessment on a '100' fentanyl patch. This is equivalent to which of the following doses of oral morphine per day?

(a) 24 mg
(b) 60 mg
(c) 120 mg
(d) 240 mg
(e) 360 mg

Answer: e

Short explanation

The '100' fentanyl patch administers 100 µg of parenteral fentanyl per hour. With a dose conversion to oral morphine of $\times$ 130–170, this equates to 315–404 mg of oral morphine per day.

Long explanation

When a patient presents for surgery on chronic opioid therapy, two important thoughts should cross an anaesthetist's mind:

- First, the patient should be maintained on his or her background dose of opioid.
- Second, additional analgesia to cover acute pain should be added to the baseline opioid dose.

Usually the additional analgesia will need to be given as a larger dose than that given to an opioid-naive patient because of the problem of tolerance. A 100 fentanyl patch delivers 100 µg of fentanyl per hour, 2.4 mg per day. This is a fairly substantial dose of fentanyl and should be appreciated by an anaesthetist, who may need to prescribe postoperative analgesia to a patient used to wearing such a patch. The equivalent dose of oral morphine is 130–170 times the dose administered by fentanyl patch. Fentanyl at 2.4 mg per day is equivalent to 315–404 mg of morphine per day.

SBA Question 78: Delayed emergence

In a 67-year-old previously fit and well female patient at the end of a laparoscopically assisted anterior resection, it is noted that the patient is still apnoeic 15 minutes after the volatile anaesthetic has been turned off. The patient had a rapid sequence induction. Expired gas desflurane concentration is only 0.74%. To aid your decision-making as to the cause of the delay, which ONE of the following would be most useful?

(a) Assess response to naloxone to exclude opioid excess
(b) Take the patient for a computerised tomogram of the head to look for a stroke
(c) Apply a BIS monitor to assess depth of anaesthesia
(d) Administer a dose of glycopyrrolate to reverse any residual muscle paralysis
(e) Provide supportive care with full anaesthetic monitoring but with no additional intervention for a further 15 minutes

Answer: e

Short explanation
Naloxone is inadvisable, as it may disastrously reverse all analgesia. Stroke is rare and it would be too soon to consider a CT scan. BIS would be unlikely to add useful information. Glycopyrrolate does not reverse muscle paralysis.

Long explanation
This type of clinical question should be easy for a candidate to answer. Think about what you would do in your everyday practice. Think of common things and what your reaction would be in the real world. The more common reasons why this patient may be failing to breathe are opioid excess, residual anaesthetic agent or residual muscle paralysis. These may be present singularly or in combination.

Of the options listed here, opioid excess is a possibility, but the use of diagnostic naloxone is a radical test for so early on in the process. Naloxone has been known to fully reverse analgesia and cause massive rises in blood pressure, causing strokes. Residual muscle paralysis is a distinct possibility, and assessment along with reversal would be ideal. This is not given as an option, as glycopyrrolate is not a reversal agent, so we need to look elsewhere. The patient still has 0.74% desflurane in her expired gas, and this may be enough to cause or at least contribute to her apnoea. The fact that 0.74% desflurane remains after 15 minutes with the vaporiser off might indicate that the fresh gas flow needs to be turned up. This figure should be allowed to fall to 0.0% before you become concerned about the rarer causes of apnoea.

A BIS (bispectral index) monitor applied at this stage in the proceedings is probably of little use. At light levels of anaesthesia, BIS shows a wide variation of inter-individual response, with some patients unconscious and some awake with the same BIS value.

Stroke does occur under anaesthesia but is a rare event. Fifteen minutes after the end of the procedure, the plan to go for a CT scan to look for a stroke is premature.

Another rare option that is not explored here but would also suit the management plan of supportive care would be the diagnosis of suxamethonium apnoea. Even though suxamethonium use is not explicit, a rapid sequence was performed, and so for the sake of this question it would be reasonable to assume that suxamethonium has been given.

SBA Question 79: Induction of anaesthesia in shock

You are asked to anaesthetise a patient for emergency laparotomy. The patient has an ASA score of III with a known significant history of ischaemic disease. Which ONE of the following statements about rapid sequence induction of anaesthesia in shocked patients is best supported?

(a) Etomidate causes less cardiovascular depression than other IV induction agents and is preferred for induction of anaesthesia in trauma
(b) A low pulse oximeter reading during induction of anaesthesia reliably suggests inadequate oxygenation
(c) Hypotension during induction should be diagnosed by palpating the pulse if an arterial line is not available
(d) If the patient cannot be intubated after two attempts with optimal head/neck positioning, he/she should be ventilated until spontaneous ventilation returns and then woken from anaesthesia
(e) Opioid drugs should not be used, as they cause a prolonged period of apnoea in shocked patients

Answer: c

Short explanation
There is no evidence to prefer one agent over another in trauma, but etomidate causes adrenal suppression. By definition this is emergency surgery so waking the patient is rarely appropriate. Opioid drugs allow a lower dose of induction agent and are recommended. Pulse oximetry is unreliable with poor peripheral perfusion.

Long explanation
Induction in shock is only justified where immediate surgery or ventilation is required and cannot be delayed for adequate resuscitation. Ideally an arterial line should be sited prior to induction in hypotensive patients. When this is not possible, setting an automated non-invasive blood pressure machine to 'stat' mode is an acceptable alternative, although keeping a finger on the pulse may give an earlier indication of a falling blood pressure.

The choice of induction agent in shocked patients is not clear-cut. Etomidate has the advantage of cardiostability, but it has a slow onset and a single dose suppresses adrenocortical function; the resultant fall in cortisol and aldosterone is significant in the context of shock. Thiopental has a rapid action but a long duration and more cardiodepressant activity than other agents. Propofol inhibits airway reflexes and this may facilitate laryngoscopy at a lower induction dose. Ketamine should be considered in cases of cardiovascular collapse because of its sympathomimetic activity.

The dose of agent should be judicious, and the use of an opioid allows intubation at a lower dose with less cardiac effect than an opioid-free technique, and also decreases the risk of awareness. Short-acting opioids such as alfentanyl or remifentanyl have a similar duration of action to suxamethonium, and naloxone can be used to reverse opioid activity if required.

Patients are usually woken after failed intubation, but in this situation this is rarely appropriate. Priority must be given to maintenance of oxygenation, and the patient should be ventilated via bag and mask or LMA/ProSeal LMA. If oxygenation fails, cricoid pressure should be reduced and if necessary ventilation should proceed via cricothyrotomy.

Pulse oximeters can be misleading in hypotensive patients, and a low reading may be due to poor peripheral perfusion rather than failure of adequate oxygenation and ventilation.

Cranshaw J, Nolan J. Airway management after major trauma. *Contin Educ Anaesth Crit Care Pain* 2006; **6**: 124–7. Available online at ceaccp.oxfordjournals.org/contents/6/3/124 (accessed 15 March 2012).

Sinclair R, Luxton M. Rapid sequence induction. *Contin Educ Anaesth Crit Care Pain* 2005; **5**: 45–8. Available online at ceaccp.oxfordjournals.org/contents/5/2/45 (accessed 15 March 20132).

SBA Question 80: Nerve stimulators

You carry out an axillary nerve block using a nerve stimulator. Which ONE of the following statements is most accurate in describing the nerve stimulation you are carrying out as part of the block?

(a) Positive stimulation at a current of 0.2 mA suggests that injection of local anaesthetic will produce a reliable nerve block
(b) Positive stimulation at a current of 0.5 mA suggests that injection of local anaesthetic will produce a reliable nerve block
(c) The nerve stimulator should operate at 1–2 Hz to avoid damage to the nerve
(d) The duration of each stimulus generated by the nerve stimulator should be 1–2 ms to allow easy visualisation of the contractions
(e) Nerve stimulators used for monitoring neuromuscular blockade and those used for nerve blockade are interchangeable

Answer: b

Short explanation
Positive stimulation at 0.2 mA suggests intraneural placement, and injection should be avoided. The stimulator operates at 1–2 Hz for reasons of patient comfort and nerve localisation. Each pulse is of 1–2 ms to ensure painless contractions. The currents used for monitoring neuromuscular blockade are much higher than those used for nerve blocks, so the stimulators are not interchangeable.

Long explanation
The use of a nerve stimulator in conjunction with a nerve block needle allows identification of a nerve or nerve plexus and the delivery of local anaesthesia for peripheral nerve blockade. The nerve stimulator delivers a current to the nerve block needle, which, if in close proximity to a motor nerve, will result in nerve stimulation and muscular contraction of the motor unit or myotome. The nerve stimulator delivers the required current in pulses of 1–2 Hz; any slower may allow the operator to progress the needle beyond the nerve without a pulse from the stimulator, and any faster may be uncomfortable for the patient when contraction occurs.

Each pulse delivered by the nerve stimulator is of 1–2 ms duration to ensure that the contractions generated are painless. The user initially selects a current in the region of 1 mA. When contractions occur the current is reduced and the needle is adjusted to maintain contractions in the current range of 0.3–0.5 mA. If contractions are lost above 0.5 mA the needle tip may be too far from the nerve; if contractions continue below 0.3 mA the needle may be intraneural and injection would be unwise. The user should therefore deliberately reduce the current to less than 0.3 mA to ensure contractions cease, satisfying him/herself that the needle is not intraneural. When the contractions return on increasing the current to 0.3–0.5 mA, injection is advised after prior aspiration.

Because of the small currents used for nerve localisation when compared to the currents used for the monitoring of neuromuscular blockade (50–60 mA for a supra-maximal stimulus), it is clear that the stimulators cannot be interchangeable. Some modern machines do allow use for both procedures, but there is a toggle switch to identify the mode (internal or external use) that must be used before turning the device on. The need to clarify this statement suggests that this is not the best answer to select.

Al-Shaikh B, Stacey S. *Essentials of Anaesthetic Equipment*, 2nd edn. Edinburgh: Churchill Livingstone, 2002; p. 157.

SBA Question 81: Sodium bicarbonate during cardiac arrest

Select the ONE option from the following that best describes current Resuscitation Council Guidelines on the use of sodium bicarbonate infusion during cardiac arrest:

(a) Sodium bicarbonate is contraindicated during the management of cardiac arrest
(b) Sodium bicarbonate should be administered routinely in cardiac arrest if a venous blood gas indicates a pH < 7.25
(c) Sodium bicarbonate is indicated if cardiac arrest follows toxicity from tricyclic antidepressant
(d) Sodium bicarbonate should only be administered if a cardiac arrest is complicated by hypokalaemia
(e) Sodium bicarbonate should be considered during any cardiac arrest lasting more than 30 minutes

Answer: c

Short explanation
The Resuscitation Council Guidelines from 2010 do not recommend the routine use of sodium bicarbonate but do state that bicarbonate may have a use in the management of arrest following tricyclic antidepressant toxicity or if the arrest is complicated by hyperkalaemia.

Long explanation
The Resuscitation Council Guidelines from 2010 are very specific about the uses of sodium bicarbonate during cardiac arrest. The Guidelines do recommend the use of venous gases to monitor acid–base status during cardiac arrest, as they are often a better representation than arterial blood gases. They do not recommend a set pH for the standard administration of bicarbonate. They recommend that the combined metabolic and respiratory acidosis found at cardiac arrest is best managed with effective chest compressions and to a lesser degree by effective ventilation.

Sodium bicarbonate should not be used routinely during cardiac arrest for a number of reasons. Bicarbonate reacts with hydrogen ions to produce carbon dioxide. This diffuses rapidly into cells, worsening intracellular acidosis. Bicarbonate may produce a negative inotropic effect on ischaemic myocardium, represents a substantial sodium load and pushes the oxygen dissociation curve to the left, which reduces the release of oxygen to the tissues.

The situations in which bicarbonate has been found to be useful are in the management of arrests complicated by hyperkalaemia or arrests following tricyclic antidepressant toxicity. In hyperkalemia, the raising of extracellular pH will lead to an intracellular movement of potassium ions. In tricyclic antidepressant toxicity the bicarbonate raises plasma pH, increasing the protein binding of the drug, and the large sodium load reverses the sodium channel blocking effect.

Resuscitation Council Guidelines, 2010. Available online (page 74 for bicarbonate) at www.resus.org.uk/pages/als.pdf (accessed 15 March 2012).

SBA Question 82: Statistics

In a small double-blind study of pain following minor surgery, patients were randomly allocated to receive either an analgesic or a placebo 1 hour preoperatively. The patients were then asked to rate their pain on a scale of 1 to 4, 1 being no pain and 4 being severe pain. Which of the following is the most appropriate statistical test for analysing the results?

(a) Mann–Whitney U-test
(b) Unpaired Student's t-test
(c) Fisher's exact test
(d) Chi-squared test
(e) One-way analysis of variance

Answer: a

Short explanation
The best answer here is probably the Mann-Whitney U-test, although all other answers have some virtue. Pain is being measured using an 'ordinal scale' here, although such scales could be considered to be continuous. The Mann–Whitney U-test is a non-parametric test, which does not assume an underlying distribution but does take into account the ordering across the scale points. The unpaired Student's t-test is mathematically identical to the one-way analysis of variance. The chi-squared and Fisher's exact test are essentially the same test.

Long explanation
A significance test uses the sample data to assess how likely some specified null hypothesis is to be correct. The measure of 'how likely' is given by a probability (p) value. Usually the null hypothesis states that there is no difference between groups. Statistical hypothesis tests are either parametric or non-parametric. Choosing the most appropriate test depends on the type of data and their distribution and whether the data are paired or not. Parametric data usually assume the data are normally distributed. Examples of tests that are appropriate for continuous data with a normal distribution are the Student's paired or unpaired t-test. The unpaired Student's t-test is used to compare the means of two independent groups. The paired Student's t-test is used to compare the means obtained from a single group of patients before and after they receive a form of treatment on two separate occasions.

Statistical tests that can be used for continuous data with non-parametric distribution include the Mann–Whitney U-test and the Wilcoxon signed-rank test. The Mann–Whitney U-test is used to compare the medians of two independent groups of patients and corresponds to the Student's unpaired t-test. The Wilcoxon signed-rank test is used to compare the medians obtained from a single group of patients studied on two separate occasions and so compares to the Student's paired t-test. The non-parametric tests can also be used for data with a normal distribution, but they are not as powerful as the parametric tests. Note, however, that a parametric test cannot be used with non-parametric data.

The chi-squared test is used for categorical data and is used to compare the proportions of patients with a particular attribute in two or more independent groups. If the groups are too small, then Yates's correction should be used.

In summary, when deciding which test to apply to a set of data, ask yourself the following:

1. Are the data qualitative or quantitative? If qualitative, use the chi-squared test, or Fisher's exact test if the groups are small.
2. If quantitative, are the data parametric or non-parametric?
3. Are there two groups or more than two groups?
4. Are the data paired or unpaired?

Quantitative, parametric with two groups	paired = Student's paired t-test
	unpaired = Student's unpaired t-test
Quantitative, parametric with more than two groups	paired = paired ANOVA
	unpaired = unpaired ANOVA
Quantitative, non-parametric with two groups	paired = Wilcoxon signed-rank test
	unpaired = Mann–Whitney U-test

Kalra P. *Essential Revision Notes for MRCP*, 2nd edn. Knutsford: PasTest, 2004; pp. 733–5.

SBA Question 83: Diathermy

Some basic knowledge of diathermy is required by the anaesthetist to ensure it is used safely. Which ONE of the following statements is true regarding diathermy?

(a) Bipolar diathermy uses a smaller power
(b) Diathermy usually uses direct current
(c) The frequency of the current is usually in the range of 0.5–1.0 Hz
(d) An alternating sine wave pattern is used for coagulation and a pulsed damped sine wave for cutting
(e) Pacemakers must be switched off before diathermy is used

Answer: a

Short explanation
Diathermy uses an alternating current with a frequency of 0.5–1.0 MHz. It is the current density at the point of application that is important. Diathermy can be safely used with patients who have pacemakers in situ but certain safety measures should be adhered to.

Long explanation
Diathermy is a procedure used to pass electrical current through tissue to generate heat in order to coagulate blood vessels or to cut and destroy tissues. It was first described in 1928. It uses an alternating current with a frequency of 0.5–1.0 MHz. An alternating sine wave pattern is used for cutting and a pulsed damped sine wave for coagulation. High frequencies are used, as the effects on skeletal or cardiac muscle are negligible at these levels.

A high current density at the site of intended damage is achieved by using small electrodes at this site. It can be unipolar or bipolar. Unipolar diathermy uses the forceps as one electrode, with a large-surface-area plate attached to the patient. The current density is high at the forceps but low at the plate, so little heating occurs there. Bipolar diathermy uses current passing between two blades of the forceps and no plate is required. The power used is smaller, so it can be used for eye surgery and neurosurgery to localise the current and thus prevent collateral damage to surrounding tissue.

Hazards exist with the use of diathermy: interference can occur with monitoring equipment, incorrect attachment of the plate can cause burns at the site of attachment, burns can result from accidental activation of the forceps, electrical burns and ignition of flammable substances may occur.

Pacemakers can be damaged or malfunction with the use of diathermy, and both are more likely if the site is close to the pacemaker. Sensing may be triggered, with resultant chamber inhibition, or arrhythmias can be induced. Diathermy can also reprogramme the pacemaker into a different mode. If diathermy must be used, risks are reduced by using bipolar, not unipolar, diathermy or by placing the plate distant from the pacemaker. Current should not be applied across the chest, and its strength and duration of use should be minimal.

Yentis S, Hirsch N, Smith G. *Anaesthesia and Intensive Care A–Z: an Encyclopaedia of Principles and Practice*, 4th edn. Edinburgh: Butterworth–Heinemann, 2009; p. 162.

SBA Question 84: Hypersensitivity reactions

A 40-year-old woman is in the recovery unit following a total abdominal hysterectomy. Her Hb is 6.5 and a blood transfusion is started. The patient becomes distressed, convinced that something terrible is about to happen, her blood pressure rapidly drops and the urine in her catheter is noted to be red. Which immune response is most likely to be occurring?

(a) Type 1 hypersensitivity reaction
(b) Type 2 hypersensitivity reaction
(c) Type 3 hypersensitivity reaction
(d) Type 4 hypersensitivity reaction
(e) Hyperacute host-versus-graft reaction

Answer: b

Short explanation
The most likely explanation is an ABO incompatibility blood transfusion reaction. This is a type 2 hypersensitivity reaction caused by IgG antibodies binding to the red blood cell antigens, causing complement activation and red cell lysis and resulting in the clinical picture noted above.

Long explanation
In this clinical scenario ABO incompatibility is the most likely immune response occurring. ABO incompatibility is a type 2 hypersensitivity response to the injection of red blood cells coated in antigen that the patient has naturally occurring antibodies against – for instance, injection of blood cells containing A antigens into a type B patient, who will have anti-A antibodies. These naturally occurring antibodies develop after 3 months of age as a person is exposed to antigens in bacteria and food. Only antibodies to antigens that are not displayed on the person's own cells will develop.

As blood containing incompatible antigens is infused, antibody–antigen complexes form, activating complement. Complement causes lysis of red blood cells, at the same time releasing anaphylatoxins and activating mast cells, resulting in hypotension and haemoglobinuria.

Power I, Kam P. *Principles of Physiology for the Anaesthetist*. London: Arnold, 2001; pp. 274–7.

SBA Question 85: Natural exponential function

While you are sitting with a colleague waiting for a patient to wake from a volatile agent anaesthetic, your colleague examines the end-tidal agent concentration and states that the decline in value is occuring in an exponential fashion. Which of the following would be consistent with this assertion?

(a) A natural exponential function is a special form of linear change
(b) The time constant is equal to the half-life multiplied by 0.693
(c) After one time constant, the quantity has decreased by 37%
(d) The half-life is longer than the time constant
(e) The 'e' value is approximately equal to 2.718

Answer: e

Short explanation

A natural exponential function is a special form of non-linear change. One half-life is equal to the time constant multiplied by 0.693. After one time constant the quantity will have decreased to 37% of its original value (a decrease of 63%). The time constant is longer than the half-life.

Long explanation

A natural exponential function is a special form of non-linear change. In an exponential process the rate of change of a quantity at any time is proportional to the quantity at that time. This can be applied to the emptying of a bath of water: initially the bath empties quickly, as there is a high head of water and high pressure, but as the water level falls the rate at which it empties becomes slower. A graph to represent this change would show a curve which is steep initially and gradually becomes less steep as the process slows. In theory, the volume would never reach zero, as the rate of emptying slows.

Graphs of such exponential processes are often referred to as wash-out curves, and they can be used to describe the way in which anaesthetic drugs are washed out of tissues. This type of graph can also be used when indocyanine green or thermal dilution is used to measure cardiac output.

The duration of an exponential process can be represented by the half-life or by the time constant. The half-life is the time taken for the quantity to decrease to half its original value. The time constant is the time at which the process would have been complete had the initial rate of change continued, and it is represented by the Greek letter τ (tau). After one time constant, the quantity would have decreased to 37%. Therefore, the time constant is longer than the half-life, and the relationship is that a half-life is equal to 0.693 time constant.

In medicine, the type of exponential function that we encounter is normally one in which the rate of change is proportional to the quantity at that time, and this is called a natural exponential function and is given the symbol e; its value is 2.718.

Positive exponential functions also exist, where the process is increasing at a faster and faster rate and at any time the rate of change is proportional to the quantity at that time. A classic example of this is the rate of bacterial growth in a colony. These positive exponential curves must not be confused with the build-up exponential process. The curve of the build-up exponential looks like an inverted negative exponential process, and it is also known as a wash-in curve.

Davis PD, Kenny GNC. *Basic Physics and Measurement in Anaesthesia*, 5th edn. Oxford: Butterworth–Heinemann, 2003; pp. 51–9.

SBA Question 86: Acid–base balance and anion gap

A 40-year-old man known to have diabetes mellitus is admitted into hospital with collapse, and the following results are rapidly obtained from a venous blood gas: HCO_3^- 10; K^+ 3.6; Na^+ 132; Cl^- 104; glucose 20; lactate 3.1. These results enable calculation of:

(a) Anion gap
(b) Base excess
(c) Strong ion difference
(d) Osmolality
(e) eGFR

Answer: a

Short explanation

These calculations will aid the diagnosis and treatment of diabetic emergencies. The anion gap calculates the difference between measured anion and cation concentrations in plasma. The normal range is 4–11 mmol/L. The anion gap can be used to aid differentiation of metabolic acidosis. The anion gap rises with increasing concentration of unmeasured anions such as ketones and urea. Anion gap = $(Na^+ + K^+) - (Cl^- + HCO_3^-)$. Potassium concentration is often excluded, as the concentration in plasma is small.

Long explanation

The anion gap calculates the difference between measured anion and cation concentrations in plasma. The normal range is 4–11 mmol/L. The anion gap can be used to aid differentiation of metabolic acidosis, and it will rise with increasing concentration of unmeasured anions such as ketones and urea.

$$\text{Anion gap} = (Na^+ + K^+) - (Cl^- + HCO_3^-)$$

Potassium concentration is often excluded, as the concentration in plasma is small.

Base excess is a measure of the amount of base (mmol/L) to be added or subtracted to/from a litre of blood at body temperature to restore it to a pH of 7.40. In acidosis the base excess is negative and is a measure of how much base needs to be added to the sample to restore pH. Standard base excess is the value corrected for blood with haemoglobin concentration of 5 g/dL (reflecting the total extracellular water). Standard base excess can be calculated from:

$$0.9287 \times (HCO_3 - 24.4 + 14.83 \times [pH - 7.4])$$

Osmolality is calculated from:

$$2[Na^+] + \text{glucose} + \text{urea}$$

Strong ion difference (SID) calculates acid–base balance based on electroneutrality of the major cations and anions in plasma. A low SID indicates acidosis, and a high SID indicates alkalosis.

$$SID = [Na^+ + K^+ + Ca^{2+} + Mg^{2+}] - [Cl^- + \text{lactate}^-]$$

Laboratories calculate estimated glomerular filtration rate (eGFR) using local standardised creatinine measurements and the patient's age, sex and race.

SBA Question 87: Perioperative steroid supplementation

A 48-year-old 75 kg patient with polyarteritis nodosum is listed for an open reduction and internal fixation of a humeral fracture. The operation will take 90 minutes. He has been on oral prednisolone at 40 mg per day for the last 2 months. Which ONE of the following options demonstrates best management?

(a) Ensure the patient receives his normal oral prednisolone dose on the morning of the operation
(b) Ensure the patient receives double his normal oral prednisolone dose on the morning of the operation
(c) Ensure the patient receives his normal oral prednisolone dose on the morning of the operation and perform a brachial plexus block rather than a general anaesthetic
(d) Ensure the patient receives his normal oral prednisolone dose on the morning of the operation and during anaesthetic induction give 50 mg intravenous hydrocortisone
(e) Ensure the patient receives his normal oral prednisolone dose on the morning of the operation, during anaesthetic induction give 50 mg intravenous hydrocortisone, and give a further 25 mg intravenously every 8 hours for the next 24 hours

Answer: e

Short explanation

Best practice would be to administer intravenous steroid supplementation during induction and for the following 24 hours to avoid adrenal insufficiency.

Long explanation

This patient is stabilised on a fairly large dose of oral steroid and is having intermediate-level surgery. He is likely to have adrenal atrophy and will need steroid supplementation during surgery. Failure to do this may manifest itself as severe hypotension. Recommendations in the British National Formulary for anyone taking more than 10 mg of prednisolone within 3 months of intermediate or major surgery are to give the normal dose of oral steroid in the morning, 25–50 mg of intravenous hydrocortisone at induction, followed by 25–50 mg intravenous hydrocortisone 8-hourly for 24 hours for intermediate surgery and 48–72 hours for major surgery. Recommence oral steroid at original dose once the intravenous regimen has finished.

A brachial plexus block would be an option here, but is not without its own set of stresses and is therefore not protective for a patient suffering from adrenal insufficiency. The fact that the brachial plexus block option fails to mention steroid supplementation makes it a less desirable option.

British National Formulary. Available online at www.bnf.org (accessed 15 March 2012).

SBA Question 88: Contamination of equipment

There are many methods of killing contaminating organisms. Which ONE of the following statements regarding decontamination, disinfection and sterilisation is correct?

(a) Disinfection is the removal of infected material
(b) Decontamination is the killing of infective organisms, not including spores
(c) Autoclaving uses dry heat
(d) Ethylene oxide is used for chemical sterilisation
(e) Prions may be destroyed by γ-irradiation

Answer: d

Short explanation

Decontamination is the removal of infected material. Disinfection is the killing of infective organisms, not including spores. Autoclaving uses moist heat. Prions, such as Creutzfeldt–Jakob disease, are not destroyed by γ-irradiation and have led to an increase in the use of disposable equipment.

Long explanation

Decontamination, disinfection and sterilisation are all used in the cleaning of medical equipment. The role of cross-infection in anaesthesia is uncertain, although a common breathing system has been implicated in the cross-infection of patients with hepatitis C.

Decontamination is the removal of infected material and involves cleaning using a detergent. It is usually performed before disinfection or sterilisation.

Disinfection describes the killing of infective organisms but not their spores. It can be achieved by pasteurisation and chemical disinfection. Pasteurisation involves maintaining the temperature of a hot water bath for a known period of time in order to achieve a log reduction in the number of viable organisms. Pasteurisation times are 20 minutes at 70 °C, 10 minutes at 80 °C and 5 minutes at 100 °C. These temperatures may cause rubber and plastic items to be distorted. Chemical agents used include chlorhexidine, 70% ethanol, formaldehyde, glutaraldehyde and hypochlorite solution. This must be followed by washing and drying of equipment.

Sterilisation is the killing of all infective organisms including their spores. It can be achieved by dry heat, moist heat, ethylene oxide and γ-irradiation. Dry-heat sterilisation can be, for example, at 150 °C for 30 minutes. Moist heat, or autoclaving, uses steam to increase the temperature. Indicator tape or tubes are used to confirm that the correct conditions are met. Low-temperature steam and formaldehyde may also be used. Ethylene oxide is used in chemical sterilisation. It is expensive, flammable and toxic. γ-Irradiation is used commercially, but it is expensive and inconvenient for hospital use. There has been an increasing use of disposable equipment, for convenience and economy, and because of the risk of disease caused by prions, for example Creutzfeldt–Jakob disease.

Yentis S, Hirsch N, Smith G. *Anaesthesia and Intensive Care A–Z: an Encyclopaedia of Principles and Practice*, 4th edn. Edinburgh: Butterworth–Heinemann, 2009; p. 136.

SBA Question 89: Gastric acid secretion

During a busy night shift a pizza is ordered by theatre staff. An anaesthetist walks into the coffee room and smells the pizza. Which of the following is the most potent stimulant of gastric juice under these circumstances?

(a) Histamine
(b) Acetylcholine
(c) Gastrin
(d) Somatostatin
(e) Adrenaline

Answer: b

Short explanation

The production of gastric secretions has three phases (cephalic, gastric, intestinal). The cephalic phase is initiated by the smell, thought and sight of food. The vagus nerve mediates this response through release of acetylcholine at the basolateral membrane of the parietal cells.

Long explanation

Gastric secretions include hydrochloric acid (HCl) and intrinsic factor secreted by parietal cells. Stimulation of gastric acid secretion has three phases, starting with the sight, smell or thought of food (cephalic phase). This response is mediated by the parasympathetic nervous system via direct vagal innervations of the stomach. Muscarinic receptors are present on the basolateral membrane of the parietal cells, and acetylcholine binding acts via second messengers to increase HCl secretion by the cells. This phase can account for 50% of the total gastric secretions.

The gastric phase of secretion is initiated by the presence of food in the stomach causing antral distension. This releases gastrin from G cells, which stimulates the release of histamine from gastric cells to act via the histamine receptors on the basolateral membrane of parietal cells. Histamine increases HCl secretion from parietal cells.

The intestinal phase starts as stomach contents enter the duodenum, triggering further release of gastrin. It also causes activation of the pyloric sphincter to reduce gastric emptying. Somatostatin and adrenaline both inhibit release of gastric acid.

Power I, Kam P. *Principles of Physiology for the Anaesthetist*. London: Arnold, 2001; pp. 171–3.

SBA Question 90: Physics of gases and vapours

As the anaesthetist on a mountain rescue team, you are asked if there are any risks involved with using Entonox in cylinders as a form of analgesia for a rescue operation. What would be the most appropriate response?

(a) Entonox should not be used at high altitude
(b) At a temperature of –10 °C it would be safer to use a cylinder supply of Entonox than a pipeline supply
(c) There is a risk of giving inadequate analgesia
(d) Entonox is not a useful form of analgesia
(e) There is a risk of giving a hypoxic mixture

Answer: e

Short explanation

Entonox is a mixture of 50% nitrous oxide (the analgesic component) and 50% oxygen. In Entonox cylinders there is a risk of separation below the pseudocritical temperature of –5.5 °C (for piped Entonox this falls to –30 °C). Altitude per se has no effect on Entonox. There is a risk of giving inadequate analgesia, but the most serious consequence (and therefore the most appropriate response) would be the delivery of a hypoxic mixture.

Long explanation

The pseudocritical temperature applies to a mixture of gases, such as Entonox, and is the temperature at which gas mixtures separate into their component parts. In cylinders of Entonox, composed of 50% nitrous oxide and 50% oxygen, there is a risk of separation if the temperature in the cylinder falls below –5.5 °C and when the pressure is 117 bar. In Entonox pipelines the pseudocritical temperature is much lower; it is below –30 °C at a pipeline pressure of 4.1 bar. If cylinders are used in cold conditions a liquid phase may form, with the consequence of delivering a hypoxic mixture when the oxygen is depleted.

A vapour is matter in the gaseous form below its critical temperature, i.e. its constituent particles may enter the liquid form. Critical temperature is defined as the temperature above which a substance cannot be liquefied however much pressure is applied. The critical pressure is the vapour pressure of the substance at its critical temperature. The critical temperature of nitrous oxide is 36.5 °C; therefore nitrous oxide is a gas in a cylinder if the temperature is above 36.5 °C. Critical temperature applies to a single gas.

Davis PD, Kenny GNC. *Basic Physics and Measurement in Anaesthesia*, 5th edn. Oxford: Butterworth–Heinemann, 2003; pp. 37–49.
Yentis S, Hirsch N, Smith G. *Anaesthesia and Intensive Care A–Z: an Encyclopaedia of Principles and Practice*, 4th edn. Edinburgh: Butterworth–Heinemann, 2009.

Index